I0438730

# Paleo

A Complete Step-By-Step Beginners Guide

Disclaimer and Terms of Use: Effort has been made to ensure that the information in this book is accurate and complete, however, the author and the publisher do not warrant the accuracy of the information, text and graphics contained within the book due to the rapidly changing nature of science, research, known and unknown facts and internet. The Author and the publisher do not hold any responsibility for errors, omissions or contrary interpretation of the subject matter herein. This book is presented solely for motivational and informational purposes only.

# Contents

# Introduction: What Is Paleo?

The Paleolithic—or Paleo—Diet is based on the very simple idea that humans, like other animals, are carnivores whose bodies are designed to process very simple foods that occur naturally on this earth: primarily meats, fish, and seafood, supplemented by eggs, nuts, seeds, fruits, and vegetables. The very core idea of this diet is to eat what cavemen or hunters and gatherers would have eaten back in the Paleolithic Age before humans started formal agriculture methods that began the first processed foods. The theory is that for thousands of years, our ancestors ate this diet and their bodies ran very well. In relation to the course of human history, the agricultural revolution was not so very long ago, and so our bodies have not evolved enough to adapt to what we now eat, which is causing all sorts of problems for us including obesity and disease.

Because of this philosophy, the Paleo Diet is an excellent option for people with many food-related allergies and intolerances (such as gluten allergies and lactose intolerance.) It can also be effective in helping to control various chronic diseases such as diabetes, Celiac disease and Crohn's disease. Some other cancer, auto-immune and chronic pain patients have also had good results with a Paleo diet because of the emphasis on food with anti-inflammatory properties. Some people believe that limiting gluten can have a positive effect on autism and other mental disorders. Additionally, Paleo can be an effective way to achieve or maintain a healthy weight. Of course, as with all diets, be sure to follow your doctor's advice when treating any conditions or starting a fitness plan.

This book is a step-by-step guide to beginning the journey of adopting the Paleo Diet into your own lifestyle. Because preparing before beginning any journey increases the chances for success, we will discuss how to prepare you for a lifestyle change. You will find practical suggestions for how to make preparations in your kitchen and family, as well as your mind and body.

Once prepared, we will talk about the steps necessary to achieving a complete Paleo diet. Some people may find that a cold-turkey, 100% change is the most successful for them. Others may find that a more gradual, step-by-step approach works best. The order suggested here is only that—a suggestion. If you have already cut out dairy or grains, then by all means, consider that the first step (however you may want to review the material in that section for additional tips). The rate and order of your implementation can be tailored to your own needs.

We will also discuss some foods that are considered "borderline" or "controversial" Paleo foods, which you will have to make up your own mind about. And, although most of the book will focus on foods, we will dedicate a special section to beverages as well. Exercise is also a critical element to any diet, so we will spend a bit of time on that topic, with suggestions that are specific to the Paleo Diet.

After you have gone through the steps to achieving a Paleo Diet, then what? While we will offer some recipes throughout, in the ninth step, you will find some specific suggestions for bringing Paleo to your own kitchen. Finally, there will be suggestions for how to navigate the Paleo Diet while dining out and in social situations, as well as a resource section that will give you sources for finding additional information for the science, history, communities, and recipes surrounding the Paleo Diet.

Good luck! Your journey to a healthier life begins now.

# Step One: Preparing for a Lifestyle Change

All lifestyle changes can be challenges, but proper preparation makes the challenge that much easier. In this chapter, we will discuss how you can get yourself mentally and physically prepared for the transition to a Paleo Diet. We will also give practical advice on how to prepare your kitchen to ease the transition, and how to get support from family and friends who may not understand why you are deciding to take this journey.

*Preparing Your Mind for a Change*

## *Setting Goals*

You have already made a big step toward making a change in your lifestyle by reading this book to get started! Whether you first heard about the Paleo Diet from a friend, the Internet, your doctor, in a magazine, or on television, something about this diet caused you to get interested want to get more information. Jumping into making the change straightaway without much forethought will likely cause you some frustration when you hit the first bumps or temptations, which may lead you to feel like a failure and give up on the diet too quickly to be able to see positive results.

To help avoid this frustration, try to set some concrete goals that are both measurable and reasonable. To start, ask yourself the following questions:

- What are my goals for going on this diet? Do I hope to lose weight? Improve a medical condition? Improve overall health and fitness?
- How will I measure my progress? Pounds or inches lost? Measurable medical statistics such as blood pressure, cholesterol, or blood sugar levels? Or more subjective measures, such as energy or pain levels?
- What is a reasonable time to achieve my goal? When will I mark a half-way point? What are some short-term goals I can set that will keep me motivated in the very beginning? What are some long-term goals I can set for the future?
- What kinds of motivators work for me? Am I intrinsically motivated—in other words, will just setting the goal be enough to motivate me? Or am I more externally motivated—do I need tangible rewards to motivate me? What are some rewards I can use to keep myself motivated?
- How do I react to challenges? Do I like to jump in feet first? Or do I like to ease into the water gradually?
- What do I think will be the easiest parts about transitioning into a new diet? What am I excited about?

- What do I expect to be the most challenging parts about transitioning into a new diet for me? How can I prepare for those possible challenges now?

## *Journal Writing*

Consider keeping a journal throughout the process. It could be a private journal, either electronic or written, or a public journal, such as a blog. Some people find that writing a blog helps them to be more accountable to a diet and find a community of like-minded people to connect with. Others prefer to keep their feelings private. Either way, writing regularly can be helpful to process your thoughts and feelings as you transition into a new lifestyle. Start by writing down your answers to the questions above and setting your goals. Writing down your goals will help you to articulate them clearly and can help motivate you as you see how far you've come from the beginning.

Once you've begun the process, continue to write about how it's going. Here are some questions to help you:

- What inspired me or challenged you today?
- How am I feeling mentally and physically?
- What did I eat today that was really good or really bad?
- What physical activities did I do today, and how did they make me feel?
- How am I progressing toward my goals and how does that make me feel?

Whether you write once a meal, once a day, or only once a week, taking the time to chart your progress and articulate your thoughts will help you work through challenges and meet your goals.

## *Visualization*

Professional athletes and performance artists also use a strategy to mentally prepare themselves for a big event through visualization. With visualization, you imagine yourself going through the motions—whether it's shooting a free throw at Madison Square Garden, playing a piano concerto at Radio City Music Hall, or politely turning down Grandma's stuffing at Thanksgiving.

## *Before and After Photos*

There is a reason reality shows are so popular—people love a good before and after photo session. From interior design to classic car building, baby growth to weight loss, we love to see changes and improvement over time. So, now that you're at the very beginning of your journey, consider taking a "before" photo and measurements to help motivate you. Some people stick them on their refrigerators to help ward off temptations, but you can also put them in your journal to refer back to when you're looking for a little extra motivation.

Taking "before" measurements in inches/centimeters of your chest, waist, hips, biceps, thighs is also recommended, rather than relying on the scale alone. First of all, a variety of factors can affect our weights, such water weight. Also, muscle weighs more than fat, so if you are looking to gain muscle, measurements in inches will give a more accurate view of muscle development. Keeping track of all of the above and seeing the progress you've already made over time can help you stay motivated when you hit a period when you may feel like giving up.

*Preparing Your Body*

While preparing your mind by setting reasonable goals and measuring them is very important, you may also want to prepare your body for a change. There are three basic approaches to how you will adjust your body to the Paleo Diet: all at once, gradually, or the 80/20 approach. Which approach you choose depends largely on your personality, your goals, and your circumstances.

- **All at once:** If you have a serious health risk (such as a life-threatening allergy) or tend to stay on track better if all other distracters are eliminated, then jumping into the Paleo Diet all at once may be the route for you. In this case, you may go through the ten steps suggest here in only a day or two. Also, if you have already eliminated processed foods and dairy or grains from your diet, you may already be halfway to fully Paleo, and be able to complete the steps in a very short timetable.

- **Gradually:** For some people, jumping into the Paleo Diet in just a few days can be too daunting. They may feel some side effects from changing their diets so drastically all at once or feel too deprived of the foods they once enjoyed and are not able to stay the course. Sometimes, these lapses cause people to derail completely and give up. If you think you're not ready to jump right into the Paleo Diet completely, try taking each step at time. Maybe give yourself a week for each step. By integrating the diet changes more slowly, you will see results more slowly, but you will also give your body more time to adjust and will experience fewer side effects and may stay more motivated in the long run.

- **80/20**: This approach is for people who feel a bit of panic at the thought of cutting certain foods out of their diet completely. It's a compromised approach, which can be helpful especially at the beginning of a lifestyle change because it builds in a chance to "cheat." Basically, the idea is that you follow the diet very strictly 80% of the time—maybe during the week or for breakfast, lunch, and snacks—and then allow yourself to eat foods that are not included in the diet for 20% of the time—such as weekends or for dinner. Obviously, you would avoid this approach with allergens or intolerances, but knowing that you can indulge occasionally may help you to stay on track. For some people, though, even going off track 20% of the time is too much temptation to completely backslide, so they don't want to risk it by allowing any time off the diet.

Whichever approach you choose, it's important to realize that any steps you take toward health will be beneficial, so choose the plan that you feel will get you the best results. You can always decide to take a different path at any time. It is a journey, after all.

## Preparing Your Kitchen

Now that you've set some goals and decided how you want to proceed, it's time to start taking some practical steps toward changing your diet by changing your kitchen. There are basically two different approaches you can take to changing your kitchen in preparation for a change in diet.

If you're the type of person who responds well to the cold turkey approach and wants to get rid of all temptation, then you can go through your kitchen and pantry and eliminate all foods on the Paleo "do not eat" list and start afresh. This approach can be very helpful if you live alone or your whole family is making a change all at once, or if you discover an allergy and want to be sure to those foods are avoided at all costs. If you want to start this approach, but feel uncomfortable with throwing away a lot of food at once, you can always give foods away to people you know will use them, donate them to a local food pantry, or use up the ingredients to make a meal for a friend. You could even throw yourself a little end of dairy and grain party to get rid of the offenders!

The cold turkey approach can be helpful because you will be forced to work with what you have left and immediately begin following the plan closely. However, this approach can be expensive, and you may not necessarily want (or be financially able) to restock your entire pantry all at once. Or, you may have decided that you want to follow the more gradual or 80/20 plan, so you could also make over your fridge and pantry by using up what you have on hand and either not replacing it, or replacing it with a Paleo-friendly substitute as you use up the old. For example, if you have half a gallon of milk sitting in your refrigerator right now, instead of dumping it down the drain, you can use it up as you would normally, but replace it during your next grocery shopping trip with an almond milk version. The same goes meats and vegetables. While they are on the Paleo plan, the diet urges grass-fed and organic versions that can be costly to replace all at once. A more gradual approach will allow you to restock your freezer without breaking the bank or feeling wasteful.

Another option, especially if you have a family or significant other that is not going to be following the Paleo Diet, or if you are taking the 80/20 approach, is to create a Paleo-designated cupboard and section of the refrigerator and freezer. This method is a compromise that allows other family members to continue to their regular eating patterns with foods that they prefer to eat while you can try to avoid those temptations more easily if they are not visible to you in your Paleo-designated spaces.

## *Sharing with Family & Friends*

Some people meet resistance from friends when making a large lifestyle change, including dietary changes. Your friends and family may not understand why you've chosen this way to eat and may try telling you that the way you're choosing to eat is not healthy or even be personally offended by you not eating they way that they do. So, it's very important that you think about how you're going to answer their questions and explain your choice in advance to avoid getting defensive or argumentative and escalating disagreements.

If you are a very private person, you may choose not to tell anyone the changes you are making and just allow those conversations to occur as they come along. If you're worried about how other people will react, that is one way you can deal with the situation, and a majority of the people you interact with may never need to know the difference.

However, taking a more public approach may actually help you to stick to your decision to make a change and help you to reach your goals. By being more public with your changes, you may feel more compelled to stick with the diet and feel more accountable to your decision. If you decide to make a more public proclamation, in person or on social media, for example, then again, you need to be prepared for the questions and concerns that will arise.

So, it may be helpful if you have started a journal to devote an entry to preparing thoughtful responses to questions and concerns in advance. You may find, after your explanations, your friends and family will be far more supportive than what you once thought. Keep in mind that your friends and family are your friends and family because they care about you, so they just want what is best for you and they want to make sure that what you are doing is best for your health. So, if you're able to answer their questions in a straightforward way, their fears may be dissuaded and they will be more supportive of your choices.

## Finding a Community

In addition to speaking with your friends and family, it can also be helpful to seek out support, either online or in person, through other people who have made the decision to live a Paleo lifestyle. You can find several online communities which can be helpful to join write away because many of the people there have gone through the same questions and difficulties that you may be having with the diet and will have good advice about how to handle that, as well as many suggestions for recipes, etc. For some ideas of finding an online Paleo community, see the Resources chapter at the end of the book.

It can also be helpful to look for face-to-face connections by seeking out people near you to build a community that supports the Paleo lifestyle. You can try arranging a potluck dinner or picnic with Paleo foods or other social engagement so that you feel part of a connected community and not isolated as the only person that is trying to follow this diet. Just like online, a personal community gives you a place to ask questions and trade ideas, and to show your own friends and family that there are others who follow this diet with success, all of which can be helpful for you to stick with the diet and achieve your own goals.

## Step Two: What to Eat

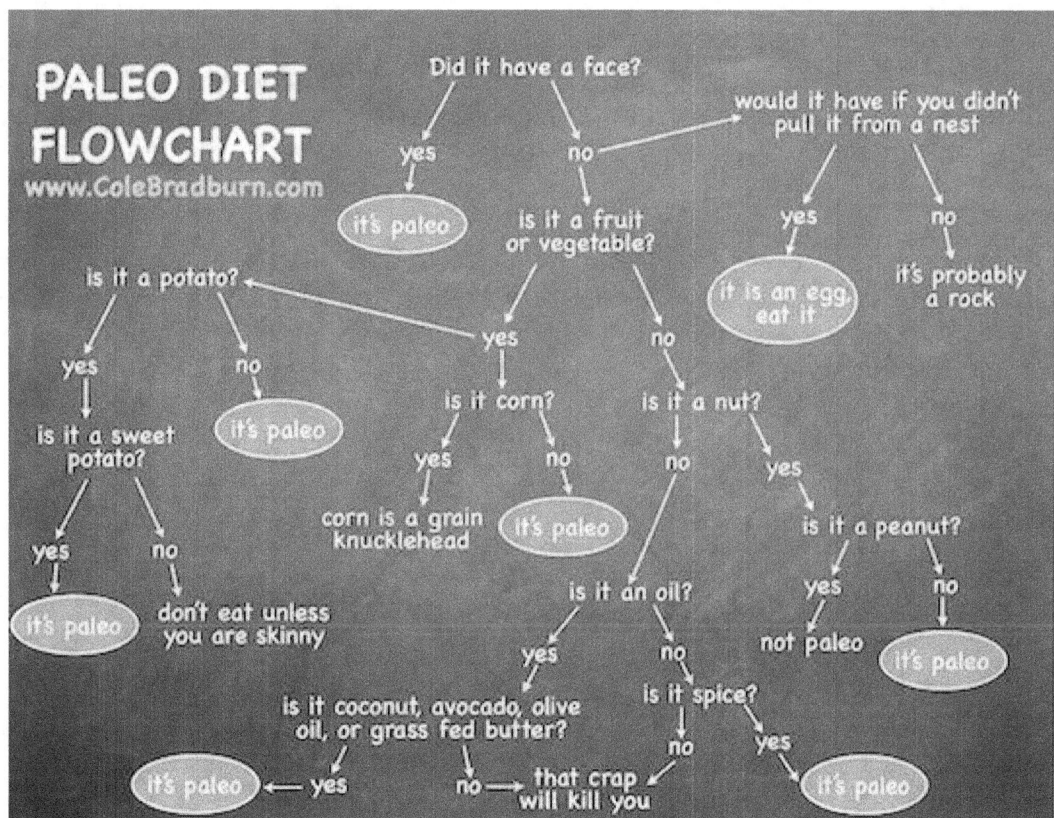

### *Lean Meats*

Meat is one of the primary components of the Paleo Diet, and what sets it apart from some other diets, notably vegetarianism. While everyone knows what meat is and you probably already have your favorite meat-based recipes, it is important to note that not all meat is healthy, and not all meat is actually made the same. So, if you are thinking the Paleo Diet is an all-bacon diet, you're going to be disappointed and unhealthy. (We'll discuss more about why bacon isn't the best choice in Step Three under sodium levels.)

The source of your meat is vitally important. One of the reasons for that is in modern agriculture, there are basically two types of meat: grain-fed and grass-fed. Because the Paleo Diet avoids grain foods, it does not make much sense to continue eating meat that has been developed on a diet of grain foods. What is not good for us biologically is not good for those animals, either, since they haven't had any more time to adjust to grains since the agricultural revolution than we humans have.

We'll discuss in more detail some of the problems with grains during Step Four, but basically grain-fed meats react in our bodies much the same way grains do because they contain harmful Omega 6 fats. Omega 6 fats can actually cause an inflammatory response in tissues, increasing pain and digestive problems. They are also responsible for the heart problems that all meats are sometimes associated with: high blood pressure and restricted arteries which can cause heart attack and stroke.

Grass-fed animals, on the other hand, actually produce a meat that human bodies were developed for processing, and those meats contain the healthful Omega 3 fats that seafood gets so much praise for. Omega 3 fats have the opposite effect of Omega 6 fats on the body by protecting the heart, lowering blood pressure, and reducing inflammation.

A lot of people assume that organic meats are grass-fed, but that is not necessarily the case. Therefore, it is important to look for labeling that specifically reads grass-fed or pasture-raised. All-natural is such a broad term as to mean practically nothing on supermarket packaging for foods of any kind, so don't assume that a food labeled as "all-natural" is the same as grass-fed.

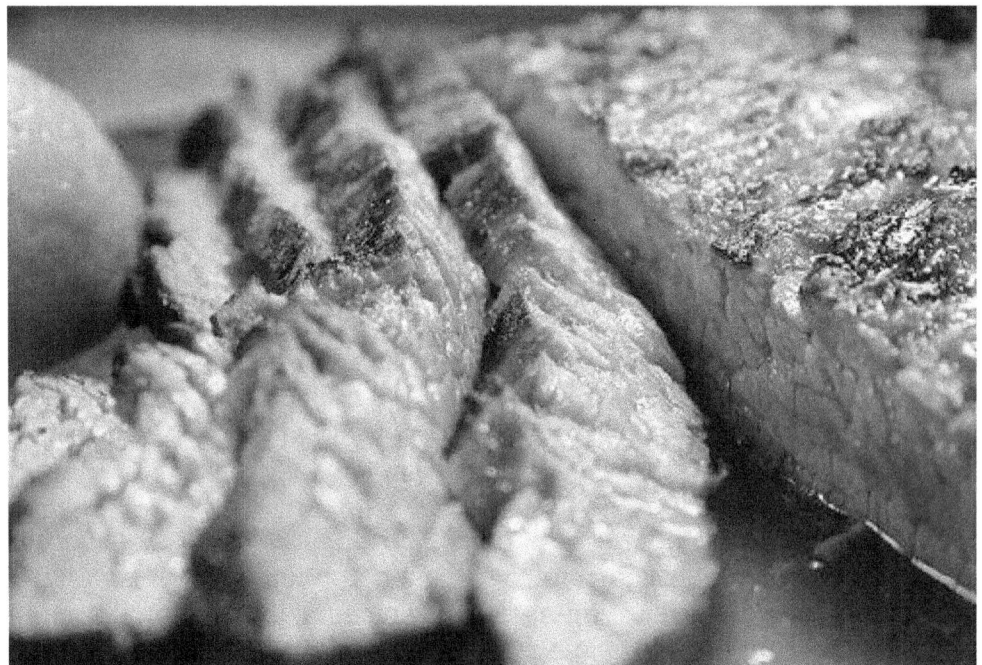
Lean meats are one of the core components of the Paleo Diet (source)

Wild game is a logical food source on the Paleo Diet because those hunters and gatherers we've been talking about would not have been killing domesticated cows and pigs prior to the agricultural revolution, although some of that wild game are the ancestors to those animals today. If you are a hunter yourself, you obviously have an advantage for sourcing wild game, but even if you are not, it's still possible to find other meats such as venison, bison, rabbit, duck, pheasant and even wild boar if you are willing to ask around a little bit.

Wild game tends to be leaner and richer in flavor than farm-raised and be a way to add variety and fun to your new diet with experimenting with new and different kinds of game recipes. While wild game recipes may or may not be common in your family, many international diets use various forms of wild game as staples and can be good sources for new recipes.

## Fish & Seafood

As you might imagine, fish and seafood are part of a healthy Paleo diet, as our ancestors certainly "hunted" the lakes, rivers, and seas for food sources. If it is important to find meats on land that are raised naturally, it is equally important to source wild fish and seafood, rather than relying on farm-produced species for the same reasons. Those farm-produced fish, such as salmon or trout, are fed the same nutrient-poor grain diet as those grain-fed cows, pigs, and chickens that we are trying to avoid.

Fish and seafood are important to a healthy diet for many reasons. Beyond the old tuna in a can there are a wide variety of fish available for consumption including bass, salmon, halibut, mackerel, sardines, tuna, red snapper, shark, sunfish, swordfish, tilapia, trout, and walleye. Seafood options include crab, crawfish, crayfish, shrimp, clams, lobster, scallops, and oysters. Just like in healthy, grass-fed meats, fish and seafood have become popular for the omega-3 fats that have all of those heart and tissue-healthy effects. For this reason, the American Heart Association has begun recommending everyone eat fish twice per week.

Some people are afraid of possible mercury levels and other toxins in fish and seafood, which is a valid concern. Most research has shown, however, that the benefits of the omega-3 fats far outweigh the risks. If you are concerned about toxins, avoid eating shark, swordfish, king mackerel, and golden bass and be sure to follow the advice for wild-caught fish consumption for your area.

Fish oil has also become a popular supplement in recent years, but the research on how effective the omega-3 fats are on heart health in this form is cloudy. You may certainly choose to take a fish oil supplement if you choose, as it may have some benefits, but eating the fish or seafood in its natural state is probably the best option. Not only are you more likely to reap the omega-3 benefits, but also the other vitamins and minerals that fish and seafood provide as well.

## Eggs

Eggs are an important part of the Paleo Diet and fit into the "gathered" category of hunter-and-gatherer food sources. Any kind of poultry eggs can be used beyond the regular old chicken egg, including duck or goose eggs which tend to have a richer flavor. Even ostrich eggs can now be found for a little novelty and variety!

Several years ago, eggs got a bad rap for their cholesterol content, and there was fear that this cholesterol would damage heart tissue. More recent research has proven that cholesterol in foods actually has less effect on blood cholesterol than was once thought, and that the other nutrients—such as protein, riboflavin, vitamin B12, and folate—are far more beneficial to your health than that cholesterol is.

Again, it is important to consider the source of your eggs and find a free-range or cage-free supply. That is because chickens who are allowed to roam and not just fed grains tend to eat grasses as well as bugs and worms that give the birds better nutrition and proteins that are then passed down to us through the eggs. There are also some studies that suggest that free-range chicken eggs are less likely to become tainted by salmonella. As demand for these eggs grows, they are now readily available at most grocery stores, although they may cost just a bit more than "regular" eggs cost. If you haven't made the switch yet, you will find the extra cost is worth it, as the flavor of these eggs is far better, as well as the nutritional value.

## *Tree Nuts*

Tree nuts also would have been gathered foods and are another excellent source of protein in the Paleo Diet. (Peanuts, however, are not actually nuts, but legumes which are not part of the Paleo Diet. We'll discuss legumes during the vegetable section below.) Tree nuts would include walnuts, pecans, hazelnuts, almonds, cashews, etc. While nuts do contain fats, they are high in "good" fats that are healthful, though you may want pay attention to the number of tree nuts you are consuming if you are trying to lose weight.

Nut butters are also a delicious addition to the Paleo Diet, which are widely available. While most people think of peanut butter, which is not Paleo-friendly, natural cashew, almond, and hazelnut butters can be used in snacks and desserts alike. Just be sure to buy tree nut butters that do not have added salt or sugar.

Coconut is also a tropical tree nut, and a common addition to the Paleo Diet, if left unsweetened in its natural form. You don't have to necessarily buy it still in the nut (although that is the best way to know it hasn't been processed), but you can also get canned or shredded natural coconut as well.

Coconut water has become popular lately, which is the liquid that comes directly from the coconut. (Some people find it very refreshing, but it's not sweetened, so don't expect it to taste like those sugar-soaked piña coladas!) Coconut milk is also a popular dairy substitute, which is made by soaking the coconut flesh with water, much like other tree nut milks. If you buy pre-made coconut milk from the store, however, be careful to find an unprocessed version, as many of the commercial coconut milks available add sugars or other sweeteners, as well as thickening agents that should be avoided.

## Seeds

There are many seeds that fall into the gathering category that Paleolithic people would have eaten. You may already be familiar with pumpkin and sunflower seeds that are dried and seasoned for snacks. However, there are a few other seeds that have been gaining attention lately as "super foods" for their health benefits and are part of a Paleo Diet. Here, we'll discuss the top seven seeds to eat for health benefits.

*Flax* seeds are known for their anti-inflammatory properties and are frequently suggested for patients with painful joint and arthritic conditions, autoimmune diseases or cancers. It is best used ground up and has a slightly nutty flavor, which can be mixed in with other seasonings and sprinkled on to foods, or mixed whole with other nuts and fruits for a snack. Just be certain you aren't allergic to flax, as some people do experience allergic reactions to flax seeds.

*Sunflower* seeds have long been popular and are cheap and easily available, even in convenience stores (although watch the salt content). They also offer high concentrations of vitamin E, vitamin B6, antioxidants, thiamin and other minerals, folate, phosphorus and fiber.

*Chia* seeds are gaining in popularity as a food and not just something to spread on a clay head for Christmas. These amazing little super foods are rich in omega-3s, antioxidants, protein, fiber and minerals. Legend has it that their nutritional value is so great, American Indians could make the journey from the desert to the sea by consuming only a handful of these seeds. To use them, soak the seeds in water for 30 minutes and they turn into a thick jelly-like ball. They can then be used as a thickener, much like a flour roue, such as in soups and stews.

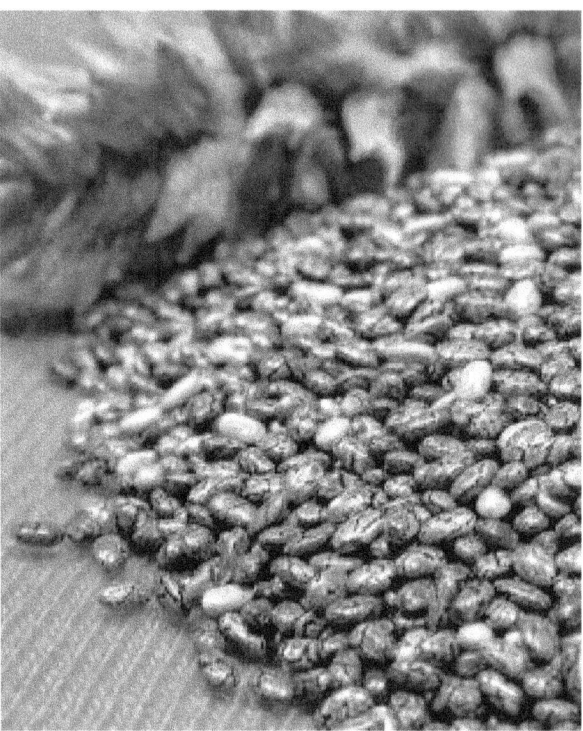
Here is the amazing chia seed. (source)

*Hemp* seeds can also be eaten. Although they may not be as easily available or have quite as many benefits as some of the other seeds on our list, they do contain fiber, essential fatty acids, vitamin E and other minerals. Sprinkle them on top of other foods or throw them in a trail mix with other nuts, seeds, and fruits for a crunchy addition.

*Sesame* seeds are popular in many Mediterranean and Asian-style dishes and are a good source of calcium and minerals. They are often toasted before use, or they can be ground into tahini, which is often used as a salad dressing.

*Pumpkin* and other squash seeds are popular and easily available for snacking also. They can also be seasoned, but be careful not to over-salt. Squash seeds are a good source of protein, iron, and other minerals.

*Pomegranate* has also become a widely popular "super food" recently, but did you know that you are actually eating the seed of the fruit? Their pulpy texture makes them unique from other seeds, and they are beautiful and delicious mixed with fruits and salads. They are from a winter fruit, containing vitamins C and K, folate, antioxidants and potassium.

*Mushrooms*

Mushrooms are another gathered food to add to the list of Paleo-friendly ingredients that come in a wide variety and are especially popular in Asian dishes. You may even find that you will be inspired to become your own gatherer by taking up a field guide and going out to the forest to discover your own edible mushrooms. (Be careful while you gather—poisonous mushrooms can make you very sick!)

In general, mushrooms contain B vitamins, antioxidants, copper, potassium, and beta-glucans, which may improve immunity and metabolism. Also, on their own, they are naturally low in calories, fat-free, cholesterol-free, gluten-free and very low in sodium, yet can have a delicious meat-like texture. Many varieties exist, so if you don't care for one type of mushroom (the common portabellas, for example), you may find you do like others (shitakes or morels, for instance). The world of mushrooms is vast, and they are all available on a Paleo Diet, so enjoy them!

## Vegetables

Even though we are focusing on foods available before the agricultural revolution, vegetables are a very important part of the Paleo Diet. There were certainly many vegetables available before humans began cultivating them, although they would look different today from their ancestors, and in order to have a well-balanced, healthy diet, they should make up a large part of your diet. Vegetables are an important source of fiber, vitamins, and other essential nutrients for good health.

In general, you should eat a good variety of the following veggies. These are all great foods full of nutrients and fiber, which offer you some of the best nutrition for the caloric buck:

- asparagus
- avocado
- artichoke hearts
- Brussels sprouts
- carrots
- spinach
- celery
- broccoli

- zucchini
- cabbage
- peppers
- cauliflower
- parsley
- eggplant
- onions
- tomatoes

You may notice that there are many vegetables that did not make the cut on the list above. Mostly, vegetables like butternut squash, acorn squash, sweet potatoes, beets, and other squashes and nightshades are very starchy. In other words, they do contain nutrients, but their sugar levels are also quite high, so they should be limited or used in moderation.

*Legumes* such as peas, lentils, peanuts, green beans and all other types of beans, chickpeas and all types of soy and soy products are not Paleo-friendly and should be avoided. The reason is similar to why starchy vegetables are to be avoided: while they do offer protein, they also contain a high number of carbohydrates that overload your system with sugars, just like grains. While their nutrient content is actually higher and they contain more fiber than grains, the digestive problems they cause far outweigh their benefits. Some legumes are obviously better than others, but on the whole, they are not considered part of the Paleo Diet.

*Corn* and corn products are actually from a grain and are discussed in more detail in that chapter.

## Fruits

Like vegetables, fruits would have been available to our ancestors on trees and bushes, although their modern cultivars make them contain more sugar and less fiber than their ancestors had. Still, citrus fruits, tree fruits, grapes, and tropical fruits are all a good source of nutrients and are included in most Paleo Diet plans. (See the section about sugar in the next chapter for those fruits that some people want to avoid.) Like vegetables and other foods, organic and pesticide-free fruit sources are the best bet to avoiding potentially dangerous chemicals that can harm your health.

## Berries

Berries, of course, would have been gathered by Paleolithic people and include a wide range of antioxidants and vitamins. Blueberries have been popularized as a "super food" recently in the media, but there are many other types of edible berries available as well including strawberries, raspberries, blackberries, goji berries, huckleberries, cranberries, gooseberries,

## Herbs and Spices

Finally, how do we make all this delicious Paleo-friendly food yummy to eat? By seasoning them with herbs and spices of course! Most of the herbs and spices available to us today would have been available and gathered in some form by our ancestors, and many also contain nutritional and medicinal properties. In general, feel free to experiment with a wide variety of herbs and spices to flavor your food.

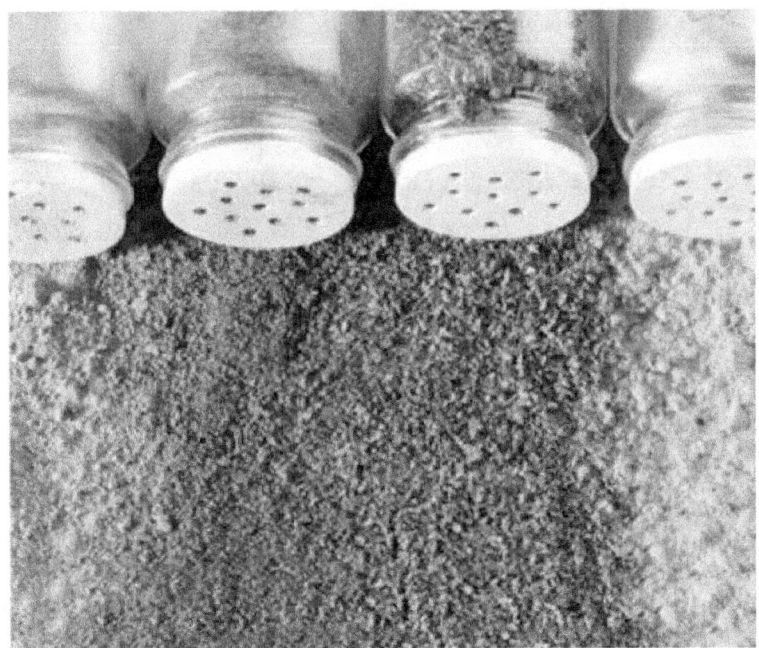

Spices make recipes interesting and add health benefits. (source)

That being said, it's possible that your spice cabinet is full of expired or even irradiated herbs and spices that no longer carry those health benefits or are even harmful. Herbs and spices are best used fresh from organic sources. They should always be used within one year, and try to avoid the generic brands at the grocery store, which are zapped with radiation to preserve them. This irradiation process also kills the nutrients and can actually cause carcinogenic free radicals to accumulate. Yikes!

While organic and fresh herbs and spices are more expensive, you can buy them from co-ops and the like in smaller quantities as you need, eliminating waste. You can also start a little herb garden and snip them as you need.

## Step Three: What Are Processed Foods?

### *Fast Food and Junk Food*

Most healthy diets will require you to eliminate fast food and junk food from your daily food intake, and the Paleo Diet is no exception. The reason is simple—you may have heard the phrase "not all calories are created equal" and it's true. Most foods that we categorize as "fast food" or "junk food" are high in unhealthy fats, sodium, sugar, and calories, while being low on vitamins and nutrients.

However, there are many other foods that don't come out of a deep fryer that are equally harmful for similar reasons. By virtue of focusing on a diet available before the agricultural revolution, the Paleo Diet eliminates all processed foods, which are any foods altered from their natural state by adding chemicals, even fortified with vitamins. Would our ancestors have found their meals in a box? Obviously not. So why should we? Whole foods found in Mother Nature are more nutritious and filling than anything science can create. By eliminating all the processed foods, we can virtually eat as much as we want, stay satiated, avoid many diseases, and maintain a healthy body. Here's why...

### *Sodium*

One danger of processed foods is the sodium levels used in them for both flavor and as a preservative. We all know that too much sodium is bad for our health, but how much is too much? The American Heart Association recommends limiting daily sodium intake to less than 1500 milligrams. One teaspoon contains 2325 milligrams of sodium, to give you an idea, so it's incredibly easy to get well over the recommended amount over the course of the day.

The AHA also points out that most sodium intake comes from processed and prepared foods, so, rather than spending time scouring labels and getting confused about the amounts of sodium hidden in the packages, it's much easier to just skip the packages altogether. Of course, packaged foods are not the only culprit. Many people make the mistake of thinking that Paleo Diet means they can eat as much meat as they want, including a bacon free-for-all! (And our current American obsession with those delicious little sodium and fat-soaked strips doesn't help matters.) Don't forget that the Paleo Diet focuses on lean, grass-fed meats, so while a little bacon doesn't hurt every once in a while, the sodium content in it makes it a food to be used in moderation, not as a staple.

Paying attention to sodium content also does not mean you can't add a little salt to your cooking for seasoning. However, it's a much more healthful choice to season your foods with many of the other spices mentioned earlier with just a dash of salt, rather than relying on salt alone. If you tend to overdo salt now, you may notice the lack at first, but your taste buds will quickly adjust. After a while, you'll be amazed to notice that what you once thought tasted great is now way too salty!

## Sugar

Like sodium, sugar lurks in many processed foods, and often by confusing names. Not only do the obvious suspects like soda, candy, and other desserts contain sugar, but more and more foods contain fructose or corn syrup. All of the above are ways of talking about the same kind of chemical that the body processes the same way and are hard to avoid, even in so-called healthy foods like bread. It's much easier to just put down the package and pick up a fruit for dessert.

It's true that fruits contain sugars, which is why they taste so sweet, but the fiber and vitamins they contain help to break down those sugars in more beneficial ways. Also, if you are careful to avoid pesticides and other chemicals on your fruit sources, they don't have any other hidden additives that can be harmful. If you are concerned about the sugar in fruit, as a diabetic for example, then you may want to avoid the fruits with the highest sugar contents, such as grapes, apples, bananas, mangos, cherries, pineapples, pears, and kiwi.

However, part of what makes the Paleo Diet effective for diabetics is that it takes into account the glycemic load and the effects sugar has on the body. And while you may not be diabetic, lowering the amount of sugar in your diet can be helpful for all sorts of maladies as well as weight loss and just maintaining overall health. In fact, some doctors believe that sugar is responsible for encouraging cancer cell growth, a process that has come to be called the Warburg effect after the German researcher who discovered it. Plus, when your body is running on too much sugar, it doesn't burn fat, which is why it's so difficult to lose weight on a diet based on sugars.

In the simplest of terms, the way sugar works in your body is like this: Different sugars (sucrose, fructose, etc.) enter the body through food in various forms. Your body takes those sugars and tries to feed cells with them to convert them to energy. Only a certain amount of sugar can be converted to energy right away, however, so if there is too much, insulin will be secreted to try to regulate the excess, which triggers the body to store all fats away. Sometimes, when a diet has too much sugar too often, this constant extreme swing in sugar processing cycles causes big problems, like insulin resistance, which can lead to diabetes.

There are other alternatives to processed sugars that can be used to add flavor and sweeten dishes in a more natural way. Honey, maple syrup, balsamic vinegar, fruit juices and agave are all natural sweeteners that can be used in moderation. Some people put these natural sweeteners in the "controversial" category of a Paleo Diet, however, as there is still a certain amount of processing involved and there to the body, there are still sugars involved that will need to be broken down that trigger an insulin response. The more you can avoid the use of any of these, the better off you will be.

## Step Four: Why Not Grains?

The Paleo Diet does not limit carbohydrates, per se; however it does in effect limit the intake of those things which we know to be unhealthy by eliminating all foods that have been processed, as we've already discussed. So, for example, sweet potatoes are vegetables that are found occurring naturally and would fit this particular diet, while breads and pastas require that the wheat or grains be processed into flour then combined with other ingredients—which are often also processed—before consumption.

There are many other reasons to avoid grains, such as gluten and starch, which we will now discuss in much more detail.

### How Grains Harm the Body

When humans began cultivating the first cereal grains during the agricultural revolution, they unknowingly introduced a brand-new source of sugar into our collective bloodstreams by overdosing our bodies with carbohydrates. While some carbohydrates are necessary for energy and growth, all carbs are converted into the body into glucose—you know, the same thing as sugar. And we already established why sugar is bad for us in the previous chapter.

These are grass family grains: barley, bulgur wheat, corn, durum wheat, fonio, kamut, millet, oats, popcorn, rice, rye, semolina wheat, sorghum, spelt, teff, triticale, wheat, and wild rice. Some are more popular in the typical Western diet than others, but all are basically nutrient-poor carbohydrates. You can get the same nutrients and fiber from other meat and vegetable sources without the insulin response that wreaks havoc on your body and causes you to gain weight. The lectins found in grains also contain a natural resistance to absorption that can cause digestive problem, especially over time.

However, there are also some grains that contain gluten: barley, bulgur wheat, durum wheat, kamut, oats, semolina wheat, spelt, triticale, and wheat. Gluten is a sticky water-soluble protein that can cause at the very least, gastrointestinal distress, to the very worst, Celiac Disease—a painful autoimmune disease. Even those who are not allergic to gluten or have gluten intolerances tend to have difficulty with digesting all grains over time, which causes progressive wear and tear on the digestive system, as well as a host of other ailments including dermatitis, joint pain, reproductive problems, to name a few.

### How to Avoid Grains

Now that we understand why to avoid grains, how do we eliminate them from a Western diet? These ubiquitous little seeds seem to make their way into all sorts of foods. Most "baked goods" contain grains, because it is the gluten in them that makes them stick together: breads, rolls, cakes, pies, etc. Of course, most of these foods contain the sugars we are trying to avoid as well, so eliminating them from our diets lowers our sugar as well as our carbohydrate intake.

Eliminating all of those grain-based foods at first can be difficult, but there are some clever substitutes out there. Also, with the increase in gluten allergies, more and more gluten-free products are being produced. However, while some grains do not contain gluten, such as corn, oats, and rice, they should still be avoided due to the carbohydrates and lectins.

Again, if eliminating everything all at once seems far too difficult, then pick a few and go from there. Start with some of the grains with gluten and eliminate those first. Then, as you adjust to being gluten-free, start eliminating the other grass grains one-by-one until you aren't using any anymore. There are also some great grain-free flours out there, like coconut flour, which you can use to make a recipe Paleo-friendly. Really, it is possible if you give it a try, and it may be easier than you anticipated.

If you are really craving something that is grain-like, try making something with similar flavors as a favorite dish, but without the grain. For example, you can still make a stir-fry with vegetables, meat, and sauce, just eat it without the rice. The popular lettuce wraps from the days when the Atkins Diet was popular are also a good option for substituting for bread in sandwiches. Squashes can be used as a good pasta and even cauliflower can work as a popcorn substitute. There are some good recipes for crackers made from seeds. And probably, once you try going grain-free for a few weeks, you'll realize you don't miss them so much anymore, and you definitely won't miss the aches, pains, and bloating anymore.

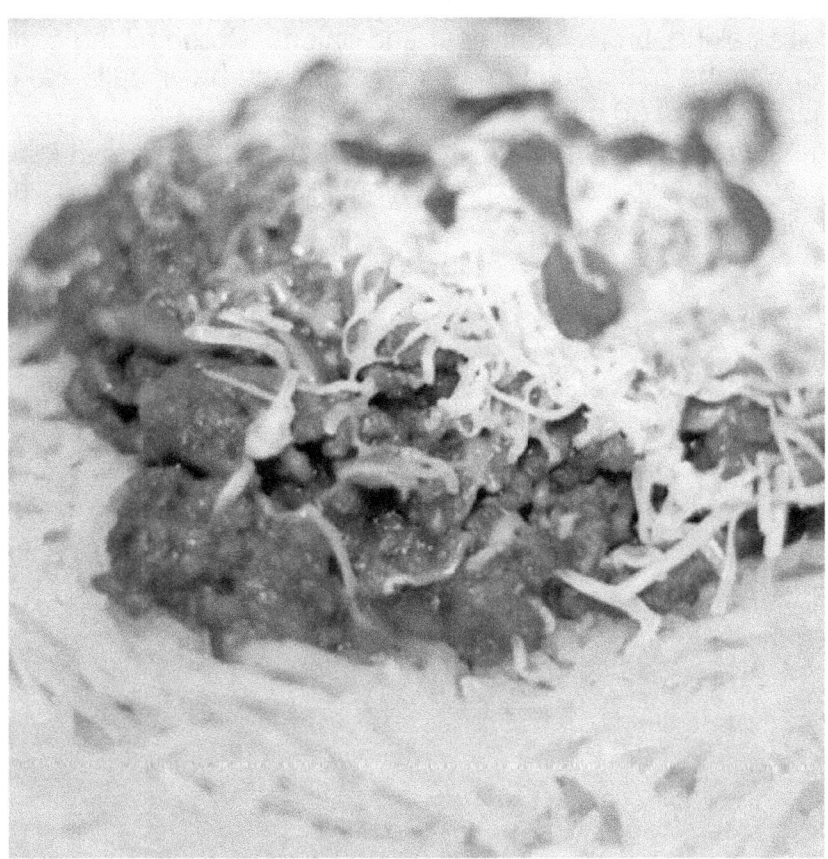

Spaghetti squash is a great substitute for carb and gluten-heavy pasta (source)

## Spaghetti Squash with Bolognese Sauce

*Ingredients*

- 2 pounds of ground beef
- ½ large spaghetti squash, de-seeded (scrape it out with a spoon)
- 1 small can tomato paste
- Handful of fresh basil
- 1-2 heads of garlic
- 1 chopped white/yellow onion
- Salt/pepper
- Mozzarella cheese (optional)

*Instructions*

- Preheat your oven to about 350 degrees. Place the squash half face down on a greased roasting pan. Stick it in the oven for about 30-45 minutes until fork tender. (You want to be able to shred it with a fork. Don't let it get mushy!)

- While that's baking, brown your beef and onions. Crush all the garlic cloves and throw it in with the beef. Add tomato paste and the basil, salt, and pepper. Let it all simmer for about 20 minutes.
- Shred the squash. (Let it cool down a bit. Blazingly hot squash leaves can leave burn scars!) Place a pile on each plate, serve with meat sauce over the top, and garnish with cheese and basil.

## Step Five: To Dairy or Not to Dairy?

Dairy is actually a pretty contentious topic and could go fit into the controversial foods category, but there is enough discussion surrounding dairy to warrant its own chapter. While some people object to dairy products for environmental or moral reasons, some people think that there are enough health risks that are posed by dairy that it should be eliminated completely. It makes sense that a majority of the Earth's population is not suited to digesting dairy considering it was not introduced to the human diet until after the agricultural revolution.

However, others believe that because we are mammals who drink milk from birth, that it can be safely included in your diet as long as you don't have problems with it. That is not to say you can drown your sorrows in nacho cheese—there are still the processing issues to deal with, so if you choose to continue using dairy, there is some evidence to suggest that you should stick to dairy forms that are as close to raw as possible: non-homogenized, organic, and full-fat. Ultimately, you will be the one who decides what you want to put into your body.

### *How Dairy May Harm the Body*

You have probably heard of lactose intolerance. You yourself may be lactose intolerant. In fact, if you aren't of European descent, it is very likely you will be lactose intolerant, but there are still many adults of European descent who suffer as well. With this condition, the intestine does not have the enzyme necessary to process the lactose sugars found in dairy products. Still other people are actually allergic to the lactose in milk. Even if you don't suffer from either of these cases, you will likely feel better if you break your addiction to dairy.

Because dairy is an addiction. Numerous studies have concluded that dairy products contain casein, a protein which is processed by the body into casomorphin, which behaves like morphine in our brains and makes us chemically addicted to the stuff. (It is also pretty similar to gluten, which we already discussed in the chapter about eliminating grain.) You literally get an opiate addiction to cheese.

That wouldn't be so bad, if it weren't actually bad for our bodies. However, dairy products as a whole are very high fat, high in sugar, and high in salt, which is what makes them taste so good. We have already established why we are eliminating salt and sugar, so the majority of dairy has to go. Raw and fermented milks may be the exception, but that is not what most people are hooked on.

Some people are afraid to give up dairy because they think they need the calcium. The truth is many vegetables are calcium-rich without the added fat, sodium, and sugar. The Institute of Medicine suggests around 1000 milligrams for the average adult, with slightly more for teenagers and menopausal women. One cup of cow's milk contains 300 milligrams, while one cup of cooked collard greens contains 357 milligrams, for example.

Did you know that not only is it possible to get your calcium from sources other than dairy, but too much calcium can actually weaken the bones? Most of us know we need calcium to build bone tissue, but we don't know how the cycle actually works, so we don't know what happens with too much calcium. Basically, bones are always recycling themselves by breaking down and building back up. The acids from food digestion break down bones, while calcium and vitamin D build them back up to restore the balance. Too much calcium can actually cause the system to go out of whack, the same as not having enough. Too much animal meat protein in the system can also cause the opposite effect by creating an acidic imbalance, which is why the Paleo Diet incorporates lean meats with calcium-rich vegetables for a healthy balance that builds both healthy muscle and bones.

## How to Avoid Dairy

Avoiding dairy in processed foods can be very difficult. Labeling for milk allergies has made the task easier in recent years, but even foods labeled "non-dairy" can contain lactose, such as in most non-dairy coffee creamers. This is again a case where avoiding processed foods helps to eliminate the problem, but at the very least, try to buy products that do not have milk listed as an allergen or lactose listed as an ingredient.

It may also be helpful when shopping to realize that vegan products will not contain any dairy or dairy derivatives. Because they avoid all animal products, you can be sure there is no milk or cheese in them, although that does not necessarily mean that they will be gluten-free, legume-free, or unprocessed.

The best way to be sure that there is no dairy involved in your food, is of course, to cook your own meals from whole, unprocessed foods.

If you just can't stand to cut out dairy altogether, there are many dairy substitutes on the market today that work very well. While soy-based options are not Paleo-friendly, while others are nut-based. You can find a wide variety of milks, cheeses, yogurts, and even ice creams that do not contain any milk derivatives, although they may be highly processed and full of salt and sugar. If you are using the gradual or 80/20 approach to adopting a Paleo lifestyle, these products may be a way for you to cut out the dairy products as you make the transition. They may also be good products to use for giving yourself a treat on a special occasion, but you may also find that after getting used to no dairy, you no longer want to use the substitutes, either.

## *Side Effects and Potential Problems with Eliminating Dairy*

Because casein addictions are similar to opiate addictions, it is possible that you will feel minor withdrawal-type symptoms after eliminating dairy from your diet. Some people report feeling drowsy, irritable, nauseated, or having headaches. Therefore, it is important to try eliminating dairy for at least two weeks to a month before deciding whether or not you're feeling better off of it. Even if you've never had a problem with dairy before, it is worth experimenting to see how you feel when you no longer have any in your system to see if you feel better. The results may surprise you.

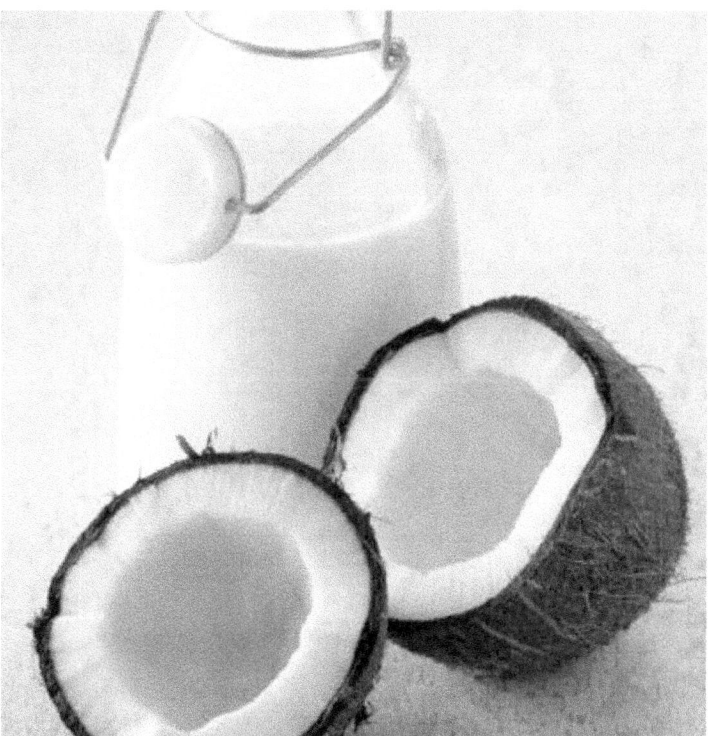

Coconut milk is a popular dairy substitute (source)

## *Coconut Milk (source)*

*Ingredients*

- 4 cups of coconut flakes
- 3 cups of water
- pinch of unrefined salt

*Instructions*

- Bring coconut flakes, water, and salt to a rolling boil.
- Remove from heat and cover.
- Steep for 20 minutes.

- Pour mixture into blender and blend for 5 minutes.
- Strain through fine sieve or cheesecloth.
- Serve immediately or refrigerate and use within the week.
- Note: Shake to redistribute oils after settling.

## Step Six: Controversial Foods to Consider

Now that we have started eating plenty of lean meats, seafood, nuts, seeds, fruits, and veggies and cut out the grain and dairy, there are a few additional choices to consider.

### Oils

We already talked about the hidden dangers of processed food and the problems they can cause. However, oils can be a little slippery (pun intended). It's uncertain whether or not they when they came into human existence, and so it's hard to say whether or not they fit into the Paleo Diet criteria of pre-agricultural revolution. For that reason, some people avoid their use. Other people avoid them because they are trying to lose weight, and oils add fat and calories to the food, although we will discuss fats more in a bit. They are good for cooking and flavoring goods to be sure, but it's important to be careful which oils you use.

If you decide to continue to use oils in your diet, you should stick to oils that are stable, need minimal processing, and are high in monounsaturated fatty acids (good fats) such as coconut, olive, macadamia, palm, avocado, and fish oils. Other common oils such as canola, corn, peanut and seed oils tend to be higher in bad fats and are super processed and should be avoided (even if we weren't already eliminating corn and peanuts). Even good oils should be kept at a minimum.

### Fats

One of the biggest questions people have about the Paleo Diet is about the amount of fat that it involves. With all of the meat and nut eating, those fats do add up. So, how does anyone still lose weight and be healthier while eating all that fat? What about cholesterol and blood pressure?

First of all, fats seem to have gotten a bad rap. In the past thirty years, low-fat food options have become commonplace while leisure exercise has become more popular than ever, yet obesity rates are still rising. Part of the problem may actually be an avoidance of fats, which then causes an increase in carbohydrate, grain, and over-processed foods—the effects of which we have already discussed.

Remember, after you eat carbohydrates, they will be broken down into sugars and transported into the bloodstream. Then insulin is secreted to regulate those sugars. But insulin also regulates fat metabolism. We cannot store body fat without it, but the levels have to be low in order to burn the fat. When insulin levels are raised by carbohydrates, only the sugars will be burned and the fats will be stored. So, it's not the fat's the fault that it isn't being burned, because without the carbohydrates there, they would be.

We also now know that certain "good fats," the monounsaturated fatty acids found in olive oil and meats, actually lower blood pressure and cholesterol. There is actually not much evidence that these same fats increase your chance for heart disease, as some people fear.

In fact, there is one group of people that have subsisted through the ages very well on a high-fat, nearly all animal-based diet, with relatively few vegetables or berries to round out the diet, and no carbohydrates or dairy. It's called the Inuit Paradox, and it was of course based on indigenous peoples of the far north of North America, who have continued a hunter and gatherer lifestyle throughout the millennia. Researchers were astounded to find that all of the nutrients necessary for healthy life are provided for through game meat and seafood with this diet, with very few fruits and vegetables even necessary, because the Inuit people eat the organs and do not over-cook them anything.

## *Cooking Methods*

You may not be willing to adopt an Inuit diet that includes raw caribou liver, no matter how much vitamin C is in there, but it is worth discussing cooking methods. Since fire has been around a long time, there is no reason why cooking can't be part of a Paleo Diet. Cooking has always been used to make foods more palatable and—from roasting to frying, grilling to baking. Various cooking methods also help us to preserve foods and kill the bacteria that can form there, which can help to keep us from getting sick. However, it is important to remember that, just like in science class, increasing the heat in foods can change their chemical compositions, which can also change their nutritional values.

Generally speaking, the higher the heat used to cook a food, the more the chemical composition will change, the less nutritional it will be. There is also some evidence to suggest that charring food can be dangerous to your health. Essentially, charring food involves burning enough of it that its molecules become ash, which is essentially pure carbon. When ingested, that carbon ash can act as a carcinogen.

Some people take these potential problems with cooking foods as far as to go on a raw food diet. While consuming raw meats is generally not advised, you may want to consider the methods you use to cook your meats and seafood and consider keeping your vegetables raw as much as possible for these reasons.

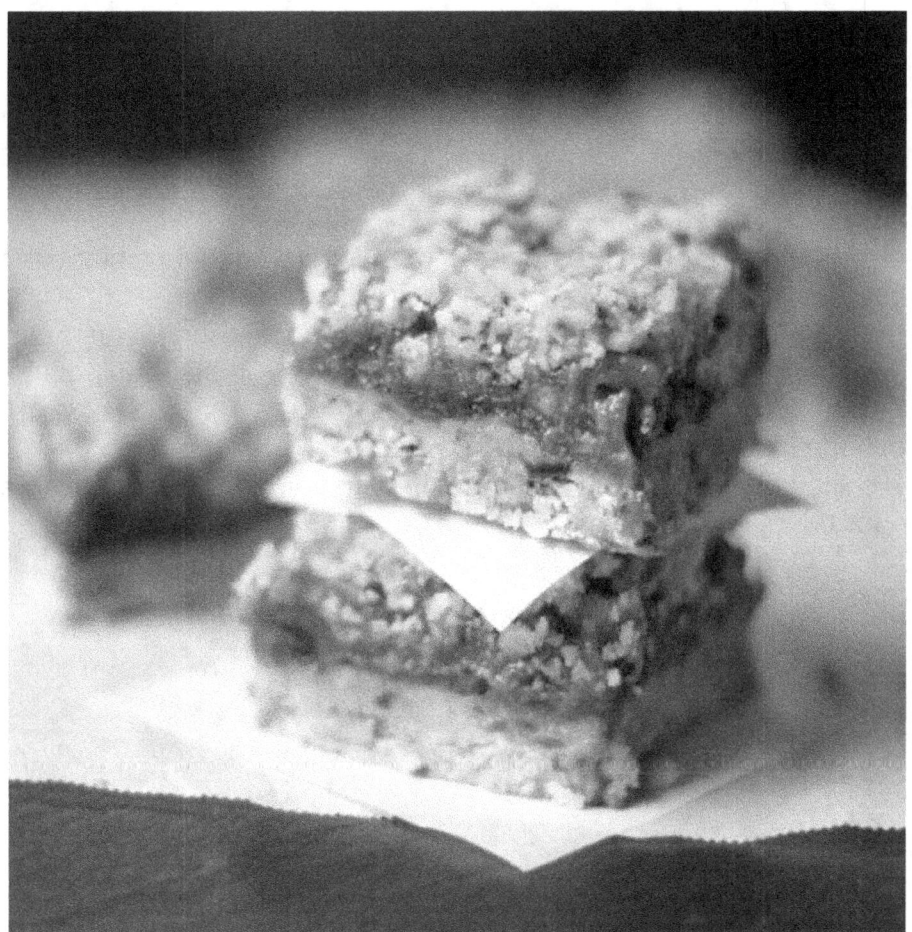

Raw food recipes fit well into a Paleo Diet (source)

## *Raw Date Squares*

*Ingredients:*

*For the crust/crumble:*
- 3 cups raw walnuts
- 8 soft Medjool dates, pitted and chopped
- 1/4 cup coconut oil, melted
- 1/2 teaspoon salt

*For the filling:*
- 2 cups soft Medjool dates, pitted and tightly packed
- 1/2 cup water
- 1/2 teaspoon vanilla
- 1/4 teaspoon salt

*Instructions:*
- Line an 8"x8" baking dish with parchment paper or plastic wrap.

- In a food processor fitted with an "S" blade, pulse the walnuts until they are finely ground into a meal. Add in the chopped dates, coconut oil and salt, and process again until sticky dough is formed.
- Set aside 1 cup of this dough to save for the crumble topping, then transfer the rest of the dough to the lined baking dish, using your hands to press it evenly into the bottom of the pan.
- To prepare the date filling, combine all of the ingredients in a blender or food processor, and process until a uniform filling is created.
- Spread the filling over the crust evenly, then crumble the reserved cup of dough over the top. Use your fingers to gently press the crumble topping into the date filling.
- Place in the fridge for at least two hours to set.
- Serve chilled for best texture, and store any leftovers in a sealed container in the fridge for up to a week.

•

## Step Seven: What to Drink?

Now that we've covered what to eat quite extensively, it's time to consider what you will drink with all of these good foods. Of course, sodas, sports drinks, and energy drinks are out of the question, with all of their chemicals and sugars, and regular milk is gone because of the dairy, but what can you drink on a Paleo Diet?

### Water

Water, of course, is probably the best all-around thirst-quencher around. It most definitely existed in our ancestors' diets and is readily available for practically free today. Some people say that there's no such thing as drinking too much water, and although there are a few extreme cases where people have actually drunk so much water as to cause harm, that's basically true. At the same time, most people also consume enough liquid through diet and other drinks that it may not be necessary to strive toward the eight-glass gold standard that everyone knows. Certainly the more you exercise, the more water your body requires as well. For those of us who miss the carbonation of soda, carbonated water is always an option. And water infusions are gaining popularity, so experiment with throwing some fruits or veggies in the pitcher for a little more flavor.

### Teas

Some people just don't care for a lot of plain water. Sometimes, you just need a drink with a little more flavor to accompany a dish. Teas can be a good solution. Hot or cold, teas are water infused by some herb or spice. The obvious black, white, or green teas that come to mind, but can also include other herbal teas.

Black teas do contain a certain amount of caffeine, which you may want to eliminate from your diet. Although many of us do like the apparent mental stimulation caffeine can give, caffeine can also raise heart rates and possibly block calcium absorption, as well as other side effects, which you may want to avoid. You may also find that you have so much extra energy from eliminating the grains and dairy from your diet, that caffeine is too much for you! However, if you are concerned, the amount of caffeine in a cup of black tea is about half that of black coffee, and green tea has about a quarter of that of coffee.

Many teas also include antioxidants and other nutrients, depending on the herbal combination, which can be helpful for a variety of ailments. A touch of honey can be added for an occasional sweet treat. Teas have become wildly popular in recent years, with a huge variety now easily and affordably available, however you will want to take care to avoid teas sweetened with corn syrups or artificial flavorings.

Basically, if you haven't tried tea yet, choose a flavor you think you may like, boil some water and let it steep for 3-5 minutes. Voilà! Tea time!

## Coffee

Maybe tea isn't your cuppa, and you still feel like you need your morning joe. Most diets allow black coffee in unrestricted amounts because there is no sugar or fat and so few calories. There are, however, the possible side effects from caffeine that we mentioned before. Still, caffeine may not be an issue for you, or you can get decaffeinated coffees. Overall, coffee is a bit of a controversial issue for the Paleo Diet, and most people tend to support teas instead, but black coffee is still an option for you if you prefer it, just skip the cream and sugar.

## Juices

Commercially available fruit juices are sometimes mistaken as healthy and equivalent to eating fruit. The truth is, most commercial juices are basically liquid sugar, chock-full of preservatives, and have very little fruit juice, if any, in their ingredients. It's safe to say, then, that fruit juices are not part of a Paleo Diet.

Juicing though, has become popular lately, with a wide variety of ingredients being used to create veggie-fruit cocktails at home without all of the additives. These juices are a bit of Paleo limbo. It's true that these types of juices do retain some of the nutrient value of their ingredients, and can make a wider variety of vegetables more palatable and easily digestible. At the same time, juicing strips away the healthy fiber and some of the nutrients of those foods when they are liquefied. So, while they're not exactly harmful, eating whole Paleo-friendly fruits and vegetables will give you the most bang for your buck, nutritionally speaking. Or, if you really must have some juice, try a spritzer: mix one part juice with two parts sparkling water.

## Alcohol

Generally speaking, alcohol is not very healthy and is not considered part of a Paleo Diet. Moreover, most alcohols are derived from grains, which is one of the biggest Paleo taboos. That being said, there are a few alcohols that some Paleos use in moderation.

Wine of course, is derived from grapes, which are Paleo-friendly. We have all heard of some of the health benefits from moderate wine consumption, so some people do choose to include it in their Paleo diet plans. Similarly, apple and pear hard ciders are also gaining popularity and a variety are becoming increasingly available where beers are sold. For an occasional liquor indulgence without the carbohydrates, choose a good quality tequila, whiskey, vodka, or gin—just be careful which mixers or chasers you choose, and don't overdo it.

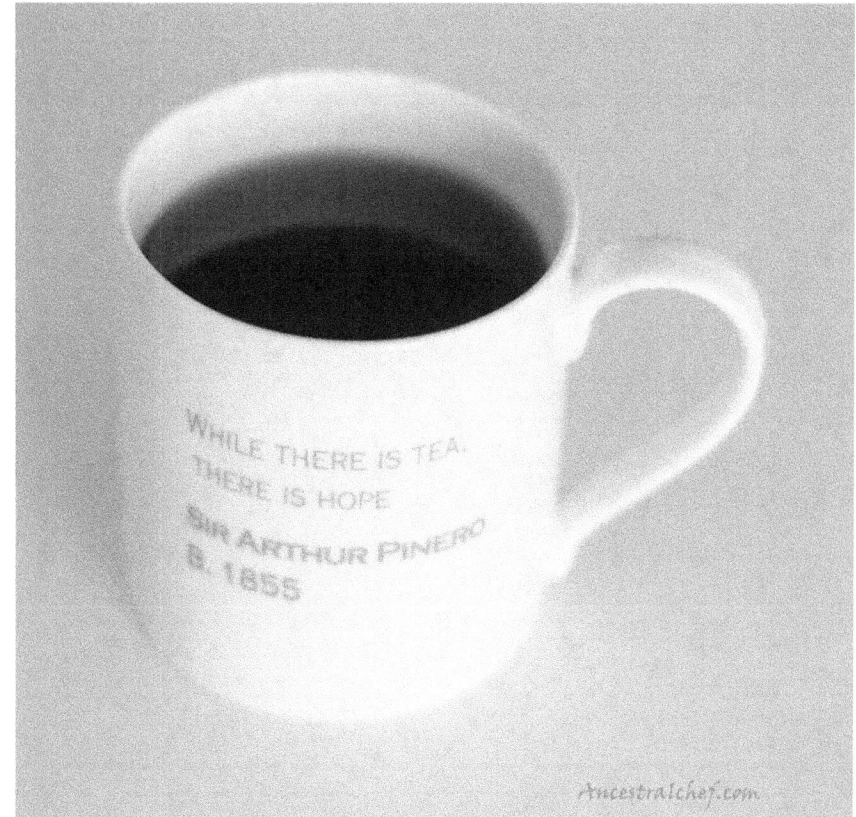

Tea is a very popular and healthy option on the Paleo Diet (source)

## Apple Tea

*Ingredients*

- 3 medium-sized apples
- 2 strong tea bags (like PG) or 4 weaker tea bags (like Lipton)
- 1 tablespoon cinnamon

*Instructions*

- Peel the apples and then chop them up into small pieces, throwing away the core.
- Pour around 6 cups of water into a pot and bring to the boil.
- Add in the apple pieces and the tea bags.
- Take out the tea bags after 1 minute (2 minutes if you like stronger tea).
- Add in the 1 tablespoon of cinnamon and stir.

- Place the lid on the pot and leave to simmer on a low heat for 2 hours.
- Let cool and pour the liquid into a large jug. Top with 2 more cups of water and store in the fridge.

## Step Eight: Exercise

Now that you're on the right track with your diet and eating right, you will probably want to include some exercise into your plan. Maybe you are already exercising regularly, and just want a few more tips. Either way, adding some movement into your lifestyle is a healthy choice, but you may not have to spend as much time in the gym as you think to get good results.

- If you are adding a new exercise routine into your lifestyle consider asking a friend or family member to join you. Exercising with someone else can hold you more accountable for going and make it more fun.
- Make exercise part of your regular routine and stick to it. It can take a few weeks for a habit to develop, so set aside whatever time and days that are most convenient and treat it like an appointment.
- Or, really make it an appointment and sign up for a fitness class. Learning a new skill can make exercising more interesting and you may find a new passion along the way.
- Above all, keep it fun! Keep trying new activities until you find one that you enjoy and it won't be work.

### *Weight training*

If you are going to do any exercise at all, weight or resistance training is the best place to start. First of all, many studies have shown weight training to be instrumental not only for muscle strength, but for bone strength as well. Plus, once you shed those extra pounds, you will want to show off your muscles in top form!

If you've never done weight training before, consider hiring a personal trainer. In just a few sessions, a personal trainer can help to teach you proper form, which is the most important ingredient to getting the best workout without injury. Also, a personal trainer can let you know where your fitness strengths and weaknesses truly are. They can also help you to set reasonable goals and help you with motivation.

If lifting weights isn't your style, or you prefer a group format, consider a class that includes resistance training. There are many types of classes available, from barbells to stretchy bands, sometimes incorporating music and other forms of exercise as well. And don't forget that there are plenty of everyday chores and activities that involve lifting, so those count, too.

## *Yoga & Pilates*

Yoga, Pilates, and other similar exercises are also good choices for fitness. Not only do they build strength, but they also improve flexibility and are very good stress relievers. Because these types of exercises incorporate elements of mindfulness, breathing, and meditation, they have been found to be helpful for both body and spirit. These kinds of exercises are also generally low-impact, so they can be good for people with joint problems or can be easily modified to accommodate a range of fitness levels.

## *Aerobic exercise*

Aerobic exercise, or cardio, is basically any kind of activity that raises your heart rate for an extended period of time and covers the gamut of physical activity. The general recommendation for healthy living is to get approximately     per week. There are some studies that suggest that for optimal fitness interval training (or short bursts of activity), are the way to go, but for most people, a combination of activities is a great way to stay fit.

If you have concerns about joint problems, especially if you've had previous injuries, are older than fifty, or are just starting an exercise program, low-impact exercises may be the way to go. These kinds of exercises limit the amount of pressure put on the joints by supporting your body or keeping your feet in contact with the ground.

- Walking is one of the simplest, easiest, and cheapest activities you can do. Just set a path and go!
- Similarly, bike riding and spinning classes are low-impact, since your body is supported by the bike, but they can get your heart and legs pumping.
- Swimming and other water exercises are wonderful for all levels, a great workout, and because the water supports your weight, are especially great for a low-impact activity.
- Rowing in a canoe or kayak can be a great workout, especially for people with stability problems.
- Weight training, which we've already discussed, is considered low-impact.
- If you do join a gym, skip the treadmills and go for the ellipticals or stair-steppers.
- Many gyms offer or even specialize in circuit training workouts that combine multiple low-impact activities.

If you don't have problems with your knees or other joints and are looking for more of a fitness challenge, high-impact activities may be a good choice for fun and variety, too. These activities tend to involve running and jumping, which puts more force on your body, but they also improve agility, balance, endurance, and coordination.

- Pretty much all team sports fall into this category. Whenever you run or jump after a ball, you're doing some high-impact, high-fun exercise.

- Running is high-impact, whether it's sprinting or marathon-running. Having a trainer work with your form will help you to avoid injury. You can also take an interval approach and switch between running and walking in a single workout.
- Old-school calisthenics can be high-impact. Try a circuit training workout that changes from jumping jacks to lunges to jogging in place to jumping rope, etc.
- Dancing and aerobics-type classes can be high-impact if it's intense enough. It kind of depends on how much jumping around and running in place that you do.

These suggestions are just the very beginning. There are so many other exercises and activities, with more new and fun ones emerging all the time. The important part is to find something you enjoy and get moving.

## Step Nine: Enjoying the Paleo Lifestyle: Recipes

Congratulations! Now you know all about the Paleo Diet and how to get healthy. Now, it's time to get started. Here are some suggestions on how to incorporate all of these suggestions into your daily life with some meal planning and recipes.

### *Meal Planning*

Meal planning can be very helpful no matter what type of eating habit you choose to adopt, and the Paleo Diet is no different. Whether you write your own plans or subscribe to a service that does the planning for you, weekly meal plans help you stay on track with your diet and stay on budget. Just a little bit of planning every week helps you to grocery shop and makes sure that you have Paleo-friendly foods on hand to make the recipes you want to try. Also, being able to look at your plan and know what you can eat keeps you from giving into temptation and falling back into old habits when you come home tired and hungry.

Here's a sample of a meal plan for one day, based on some of the recipes in this book. More resources for recipes and where you can find subscriptions for lesson plans are included in the resources section.

- *Breakfast:* Paleo Pancakes with blueberries, bacon, and black coffee
- *Lunch:* Spicy Asian Lettuce Wraps with BBQ Kale Chips and Apple Tea
- *Snack:* Almond-Stuffed Date Bites
- *Dinner:* Paleo Skillet Steak and Onions, Mashed "Potato" Cauliflower, and Rainbow Roasted Carrots with red wine
- *Dessert:* Orange Chocolate "Cheese" Cake

### *Main dishes*

Here are just a few examples of main dishes to get you started. Included are faux-grain pancakes for breakfast, plus an Asian-style recipe that uses lettuce instead of a wrap. A traditional steak-and-onion and seafood entrée give you options for two separate evenings plus a surf-and-turf leftover night!

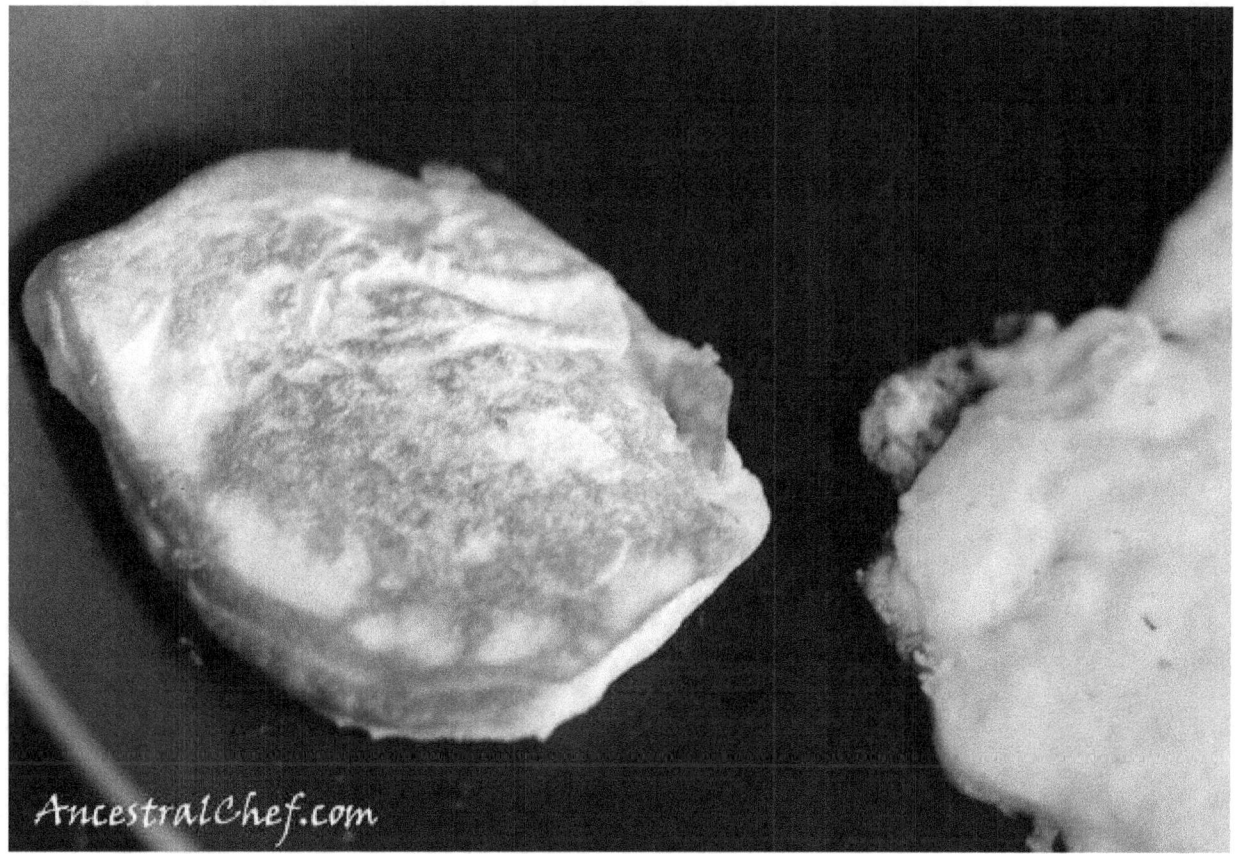

AncestralChef.com

With nut flours, you can even make Paleo pancakes. (<u>source</u>)

## Paleo Pancakes

*Ingredients*

- 4 eggs
- 1/2 cup coconut flour
- 1 cup coconut milk (from the cans, not the cartons – make sure it doesn't have added sugar and it isn't the "light" stuff. Also shake the can before opening as the cream and the water separates.)
- 2 teaspoons vanilla extract (make sure you buy a brand that has no added sugar)
- sweetener of your choice (optional)
- 1 teaspoon baking soda
- coconut oil or butter for cooking

*Instructions*

- Beat the eggs; add in the coconut flour, coconut milk, vanilla, baking soda, and your choice of sweetener. Mix well.
- To cook these pancakes, you can use a griddle or a frying pan. Put some coconut oil into the pan to grease it and put the pan on low heat.

- Ladle some of the batter into the pan (to form a 3 inch diameter circle). The pancake should be thick so don't try to make the batter spread out. If you're using a large enough frying pan, you can cook 3 or 4 pancakes at the same time.
- Cook for 2 minutes and then flip. Continue cooking and flipping until both sides are brown.
- The pancakes are a bit dry by themselves, so have it with some butter or coconut oil or else some fruit.

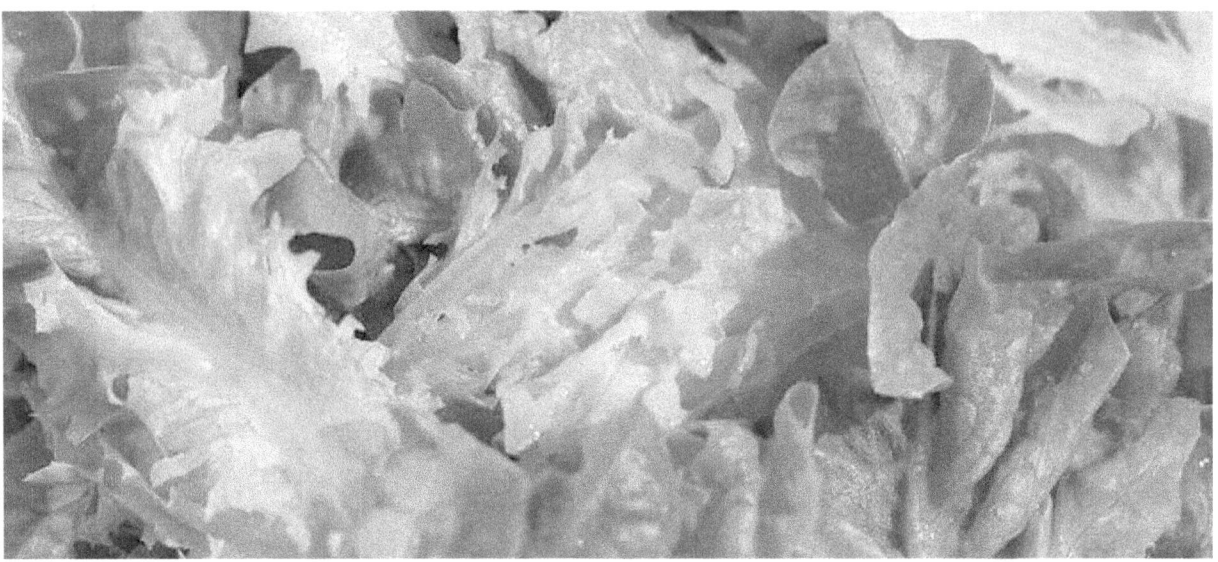

Lettuce is a good alternative to a carb-filled wrap for Paleo eaters. (source)

## Spicy Asian Lettuce Wraps

Ingredients

- 1/2 pound sirloin or flank steak cut into thin strips
- 1 tbs coconut oil
- 1/2 medium red bell pepper, chopped
- 1 cup celery, chopped
- 2 tsp ginger, minced
- 2 cloves garlic, minced
- 1 tbs coconut aminos
- 1 tbs white vinegar
- 1 tsp red pepper flakes
- 1/2 tsp cayenne pepper
- 2 tbs coarsely chopped cashews
- 2 green onions, thinly sliced
- 4 large iceberg or romaine lettuce leaves

Instructions

- Add oil to a wok or large skillet over medium heat. Sauté the red pepper flakes, garlic, and ginger, briefly, before adding the steak strips, red bell pepper, and celery.
- Cook and stir for 3-5 minutes until the steak is fully browned on the outside.
- Add the coconut aminos, vinegar, and cayenne pepper. Continue to cook and stir for about a minute.
- Add the cashews and green onions, and cook until the steak is done.
- Spoon equal portions of the mixture onto the lettuce leaves. Fold or roll the lettuce so that the mixture can be eaten by hand.

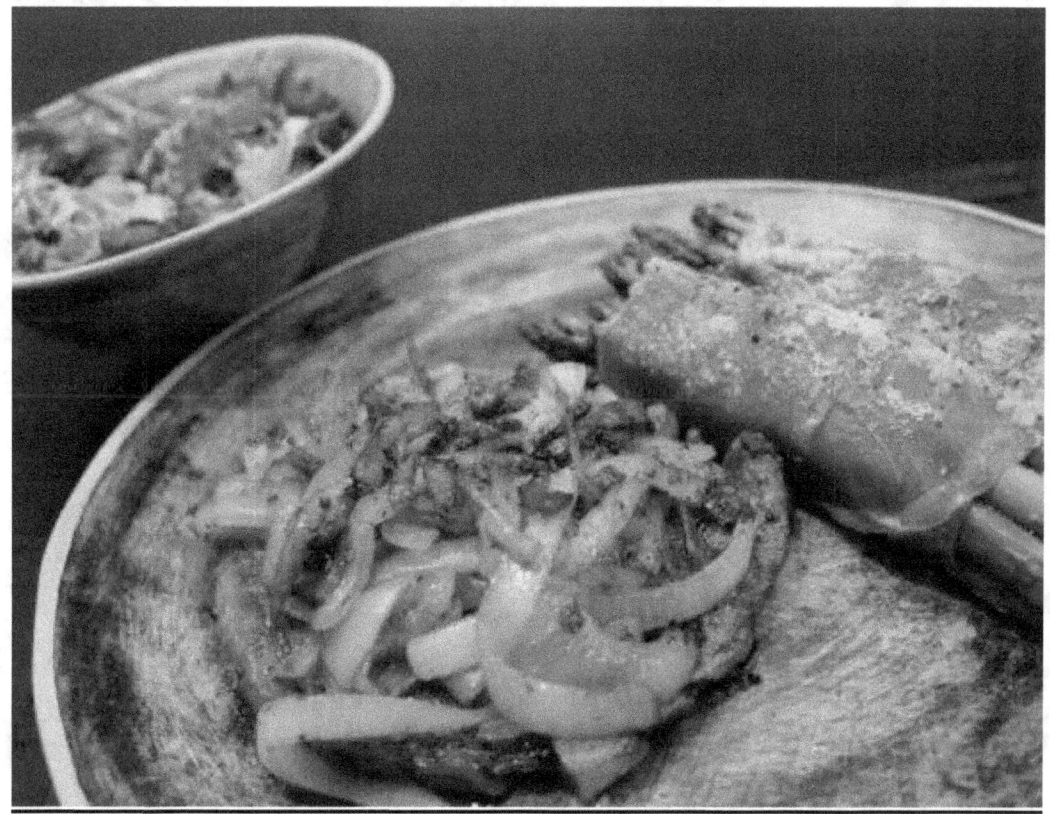

A beautiful steak with onions, asparagus wrapped in prosciutto, and a salad are a complete Paleo meal. (source)

## Paleo Skillet Steak with Onions

*Ingredients*

- 1 sirloin steak
- 1 onion, sliced
- 1 garlic, sliced
- extra virgin olive oil
- coarse ground pepper
- coarse sea salt

*Instructions*

- Season the steak with salt and pepper and marinate in olive oil for at least 30 minutes.
- Add a couple turns of olive oil to the skillet with medium high heat and add sliced onion and garlic. Cook until onions are soft but not brown, then add the meat.
- Cook the steak with the onions and garlic until it reaches your preferred level of doneness. I like mine well done, so after it's browned well on both sides, I cut a bit to check that it's cooked through and there's no more red. Meanwhile, when the onions and garlic get browned, scoop them up and put them on top of the steak (or remove and set aside if you prefer) to keep them from burning.
- Then serve with vegetables and enjoy!

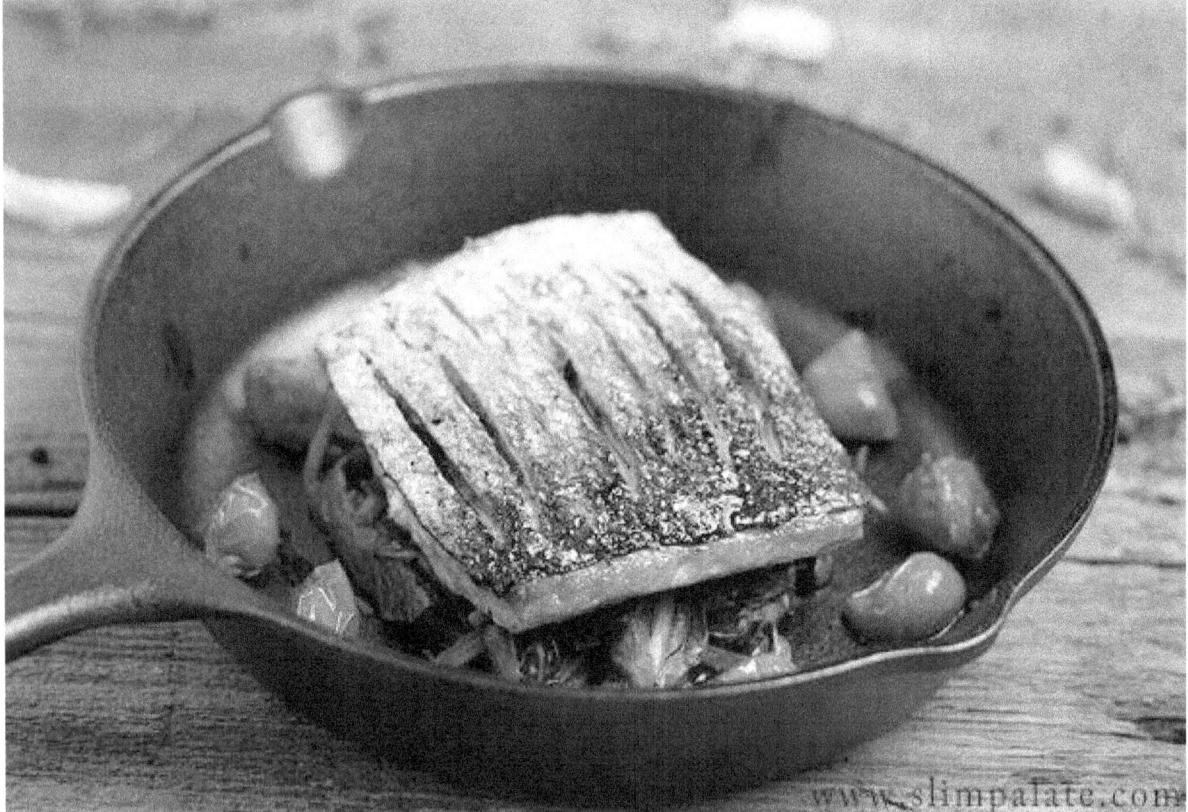
Here is a beautifully elegant and simple salmon dish. (source)

*Crispy Skin Salmon*

*Ingredients*

- 1 1/2 lb salmon filet skin on
- 2 cloves garlic

- 3 sprigs fresh thyme
- salt and pepper to taste
- 1 tablespoon avocado oil or macadamia nut oil plus a little extra for brushing

*Instructions*

- Take salmon filet and cut into individual portions.
- Flip the salmon over skin side up, firmly hold the sides of the filet and curl it upward by pressing the sides slightly in. Carefully score the skin across by slicing your knife through the skin about a ½-inch deep. (Be sure to do this just across the top of the skin, but do not slice all the way through the fish like you are going to cut it in half. Try to keep the scores about a ¼-inch apart—the closer the scores, the crispier the skin.)
- Once each filet is scored, take the leaves off your thyme and mince with your garlic.
- Sprinkle in a little bit of salt, fresh cracked black pepper, and thyme/garlic mixture in between each slit of each score.
- In a medium-sized pan heat avocado oil over medium high heat and wait for the pan to get hot. While you're waiting for the pan to get hot, lightly brush the top of each salmon skin with avocado oil to prevent any sticking. (Be careful not to rub out any of the herb mixture in the slits.)
- Once the pan is hot, place the salmon in the pan facing away from you so you don't splash hot oil on yourself. Very lightly press down for a second—just enough to make sure it's evenly distributed across the pan for an even sear. (Take care not to overcrowd the pan as you may need to do the salmon in batches.)
- Let the salmon cook for 2-4 minutes on the skin, or until the salmon has turned a milky pink about 2/3 the way up the salmon.
- Carefully slide spatula under salmon, being careful not to rip the skin, and flip. Cook on the other side for 2-3 more minutes or until salmon is cooked all the way through.
- Serve with your choice of veggies.

## Side dishes

Main dishes are important, of course, but what kinds of sides can be eaten on Paleo Diet? Try a few of these suggestions.

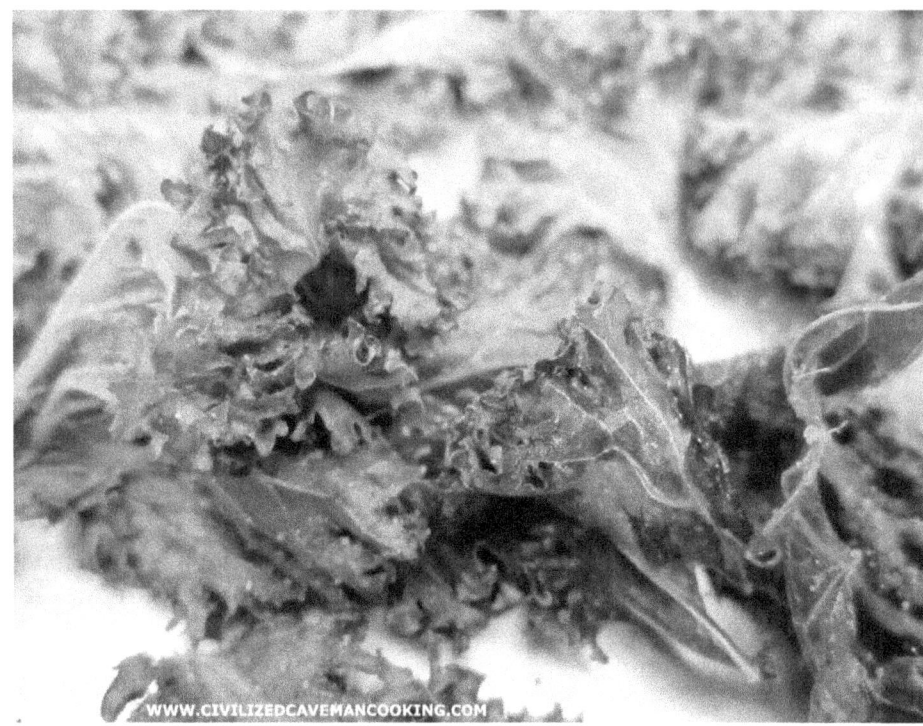

Instead of carb-laden potato chips, try yummy BBQ kale chips! (source)

## BBQ Kale Chips

*Ingredients*

- 3 large handfuls of kale
- 2 tbsp extra virgin olive oil
- 1 tsp sea salt
- 1/4 tsp smoked paprika
- 1/4 tsp granulated garlic

*Instructions*

- Preheat your oven to 350 Degrees Fahrenheit.
- Remove all of your kale leaves from the stalk and wash well.
- Once they are all washed, dry them over and over again. They need to be bone dry to get the best results. If you have a salad spinner, now is the time to use it. If not, you are going to be using lots and lots of paper towels.
- Place all of your dry kale in a mixing bowl and coat with all of your extra virgin olive oil.
- Once coated, use 1/2 tsp of sea salt and sprinkle all over.
- Line a baking sheet with aluminum foil and place all of your kale on the sheet.

- Place in the oven and bake for 12-15 minutes, or until the chips are crispy. If you let them cook too long, they will not taste good, so don't burn them. Check them often after the 10 minute mark.
- Combine the paprika, garlic, and remaining sea salt in a small bowl. At the 10 minute mark, remove your kale from the oven and sprinkle with this mixture.
- Place back in the oven and continue cooking until done.

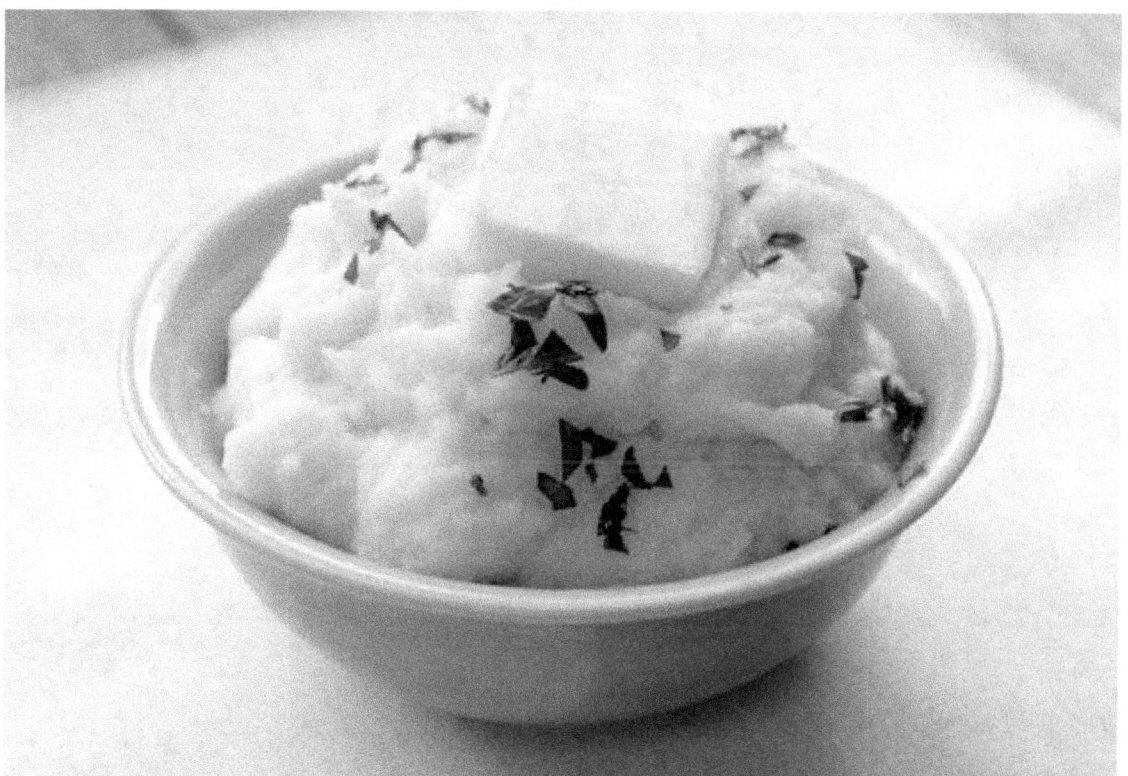

Don't worry about what to serve at Thanksgiving with this mashed potato substitute.
(source)

## Mashed "Potato" Cauliflower

*Ingredients*

- 2 heads cauliflower, washed and cut into large pieces
- 2 tablespoons soy-free butter spread or olive oil
- ½ teaspoon sea salt

*Instructions*

- Steam the cauliflower pieces until very tender
- Puree cauliflower in a food processor, add in buttery spread and salt
- Reheat in a casserole dish in the oven at 350° for 20 minutes

- serve

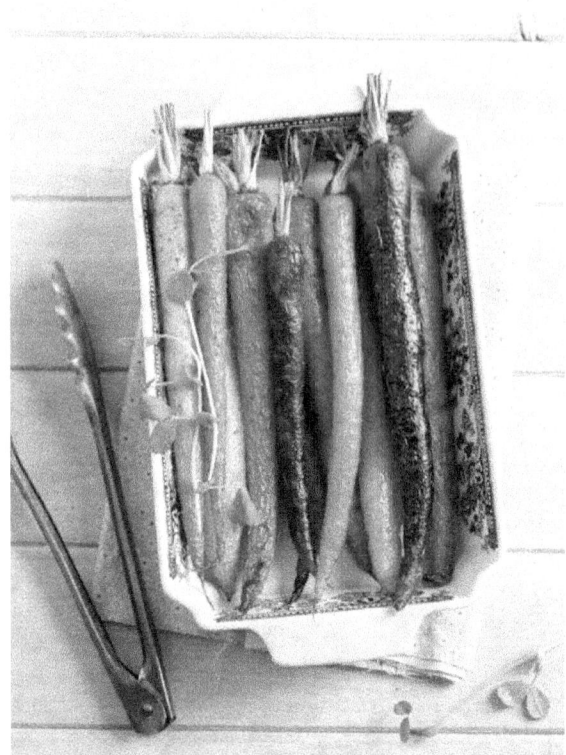

Roasted carrots like these make a beautiful side dish. (source)

## Rainbow Roasted Carrots

*Ingredients*

- 2 bunches rainbow carrots (the dark ones above are purple, not burned)
- extra virgin olive oil
- sea salt
- fresh ground black pepper
- garlic powder

*Instructions*

- Set the oven to 400 degrees.
- Cut the tops to about 1 inch and scrub the carrots well. Set them on a kitchen towel to dry.
- When they are dry add them to a sheet.
- Drizzle with a little oil and sprinkle with salt, pepper and garlic (I like to go lighter on the garlic). Toss to coat.

- Cover the top with another sheet turned upside down so that the carrots steam inside. Note: This would also work in a Dutch oven that has a lid, if you have one to fit the whole carrots.
- Bake covered for 30 minutes. Note: Some of my carrots were much thinner than the rest, so I held them back for the first 20 minutes of baking, then added them. Otherwise they would have been mush.
- Remove the top and roast uncovered for about 20 minutes more.

## Snacks

Sometimes we get hungry in between meals, and the Paleo Diet allows for all the Paleo snacks you want. Try a few of these when you're out and about or it's not quite time for dinner.

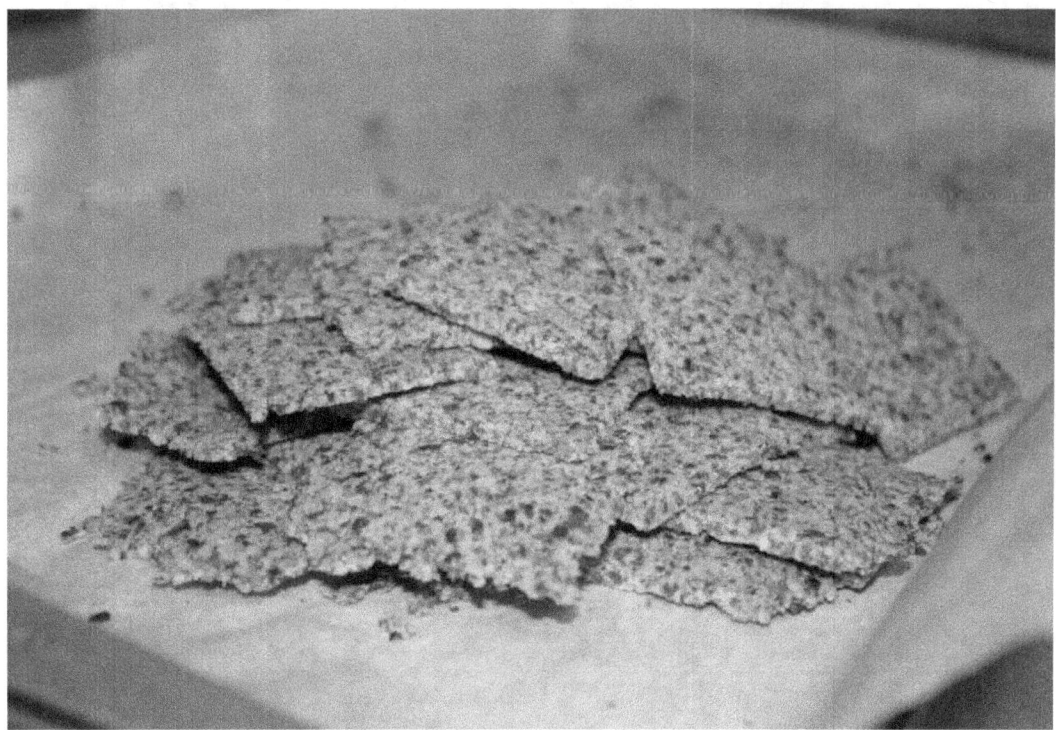

Life just wouldn't be the same without a few crackers. (source)

## Almond Crackers

### Ingredients

- 1 cup almond pulp (you can use the leftover from making your own almond milk or blanched almond meal and ¼ cup of water)
- 2 tablespoons flaxseed meal
- 1 tablespoon sesame seed oil

- ½ teaspoon salt

*Instructions*

- Combine all ingredients in a large bowl.
- Roll dough into a ball, press between 2 sheets of parchment paper and roll to ¼ inch thickness.
- Remove top piece of parchment paper.
- Transfer the bottom piece with rolled out dough onto baking sheet.
- Cut dough into 2-inch squares with a knife or pizza cutter.
- Bake at the lowest setting for around 20 hours, or until crunchy.
- Let crackers come to room temperature on baking sheet, then serve.

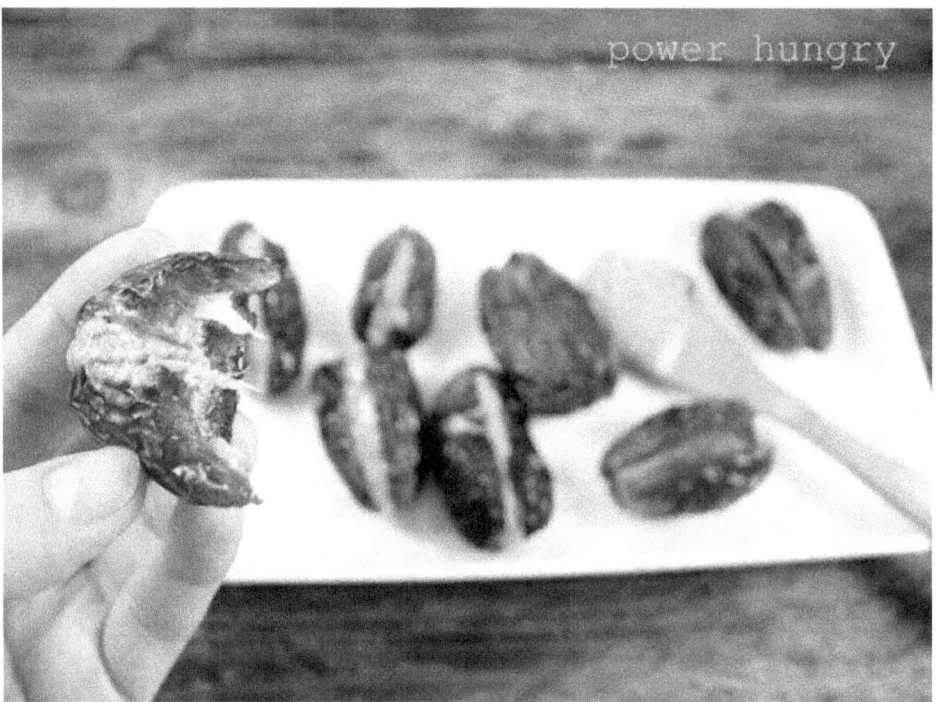

This delicious snack would work well as an appetizer, salad topper, or dessert. (source)

## *Almond-Stuffed Date Bites*

*Ingredients*

- whole pitted dates (preferably gooey-soft, unctuous ones, like Medjool)
- natural almond butter (or other nut or seed butter, like cashew, sunflower or hemp)

*Instructions*

- Open one date (You can use your fingers, but if you are a precision person, use a knife).
- Use fingers to open up a date, creating a pocket for your stuffing.
- Scoop a generous teaspoon of nut/seed butter inside date.
- Close date.
- Eat, and/or continue the process with as many dates as you like. These are delicious immediately, but the dates are even better if you chill them in an airtight container for at least 1-2 hours until the nut butter is firm (the beauty of natural nut and seeds butters is they firm up when cold).

## Desserts

Life just wouldn't be as sweet without dessert. While sugars are limited on a Paleo Diet, there are still desserts, including chocolate. Milk chocolate is not included, of course, but cocoa powder may be added to a variety of foods. And even though most desserts aren't calorie-free, you can reward yourself occasionally for staying the course. Here is just one amazing way you can enjoy dessert on the Paleo Diet.

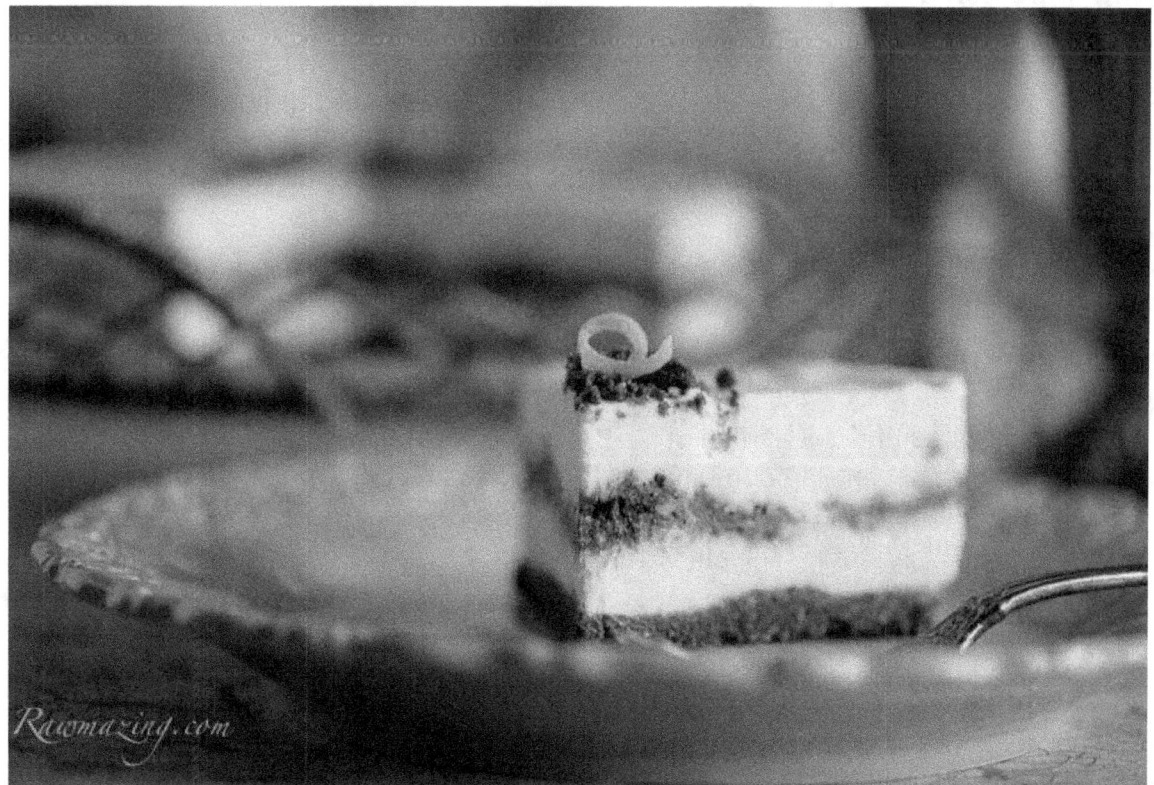

Too good to be true? This orange chocolate "cheese" cake is Paleo-friendly and raw.
(source)

*Orange Chocolate "Cheese" Cake*

**Crust Ingredients**

- 1/2 cup almonds
- 1/2 cup pecans
- 4 dates, soaked until soft
- 1/4 cup cacao powder

**Crust Instructions**

- Place almonds and pecans in food processor and process until finely chopped.
- Add dates and cacao. Process until well blended. Mixture should stick together when you pinch it.
- Press 2/3 of the mixture into the bottom of a 7-inch spring form pan lined with parchment paper. Make sure you press it well.
- Set the remaining 1/3 mixture aside to use for filling layer or to sprinkle on top.

**Filling Ingredients**

- 1/2 cup orange zest
- 2 cups cashews, soaked until soft (4+ hours), rinsed and drained well
- 1 1/4 cup coconut oil, melted
- 1 cup fresh orange juice (approximately 3 oranges, depending how juicy they are)
- 2/3 cup raw agave nectar
- 1 tablespoon fresh grated ginger

**Filling Instructions**

- Zest oranges and set aside.
- In high-speed blender, combine cashews, coconut oil, orange juice and raw agave nectar. Blend until smooth.
- Add zest and ginger. Pulse just to combine.
- Pour over crust.
- Refrigerate overnight.
- Top with remaining crust.

**Chef's Note**: If you want to use the crust as a layer (like photo), you will need to pour half the filling mixture into the pan and place it in the freezer for a bit (DO NOT LET FREEZE) to let it set up. Sprinkle crust over bottom layer then carefully pour in the remaining filling mixture.

## Step Ten: Enjoying the Paleo Lifestyle: Eating Out

Now that you know about all the amazing Paleo foods you can eat, you may be a little afraid to leave your own kitchen. Making your own food is certainly healthy, and the best way to maintain control over what you put into your body, but sometimes you have to leave the comforts of home. Here are a few tips as you venture out into the world as a Paleo.

### *Work*

Because your work environment is probably already a place that you know well, planning to incorporate your Paleo lifestyle into your working lifestyle need not be difficult. The easiest way to navigate work is to bring along your own food, if you don't already. Plan your lunches ahead of time with a meal plan, or just take leftovers from your own cooking the night before. If you have a workplace cafeteria or have to take clients out for lunch often, you may want to skip ahead to the suggestions for managing restaurant meals. Taking healthy Paleo snacks and drinks along with you will also help you to avoid temptations and prevent you from being unnecessarily derailed. Also, planning for how you will address concerns from friends and family can help you to answer questions coworkers may have as well. A little planning can make the transition much smoother.

### *Restaurants*

Restaurants can be difficult to manage for anyone with dietary restrictions, even self-imposed ones. Just like with other situations we have discussed, a little planning can go a long way toward successfully navigating a restaurant meal. Most restaurants now post their menus online, so if you know you will be going out, choosing what you will eat before getting there can help you to make better choices and avoid getting derailed by temptations that sound or look good when you get there.

Some restaurant menus are going to better than others, so if you have choice, try to avoid places with grain-heavy menus, such as Italian restaurants. Fast food restaurants should obviously be avoided as much as possible. You can always special order items off the menu though by asking for a dish without the rice or hold the bread. And there are very, very few menus that don't have at least a salad you can order if all else fails. Water is always available, too, and will usually save you money on the bill as well.

### *Social Occasions*

Sometimes the places we feel we have the least control over our food choices are during social occasions. We may go to a friend or family member's house for dinner or be invited to a party, only to find that all of the foods contain cheese or copious amounts of grains. There are a few things you can do in these situations to maintain your relationships and your diet.

First of all, you can always offer to bring a dish along. Most people are curious about different diets and would be more than happy to try whatever it is that fits your diet as long as it doesn't conflict with theirs (so maybe don't bring steak to a vegan's party.) If you're not sure what will be available and you can't bring your own dish, fill up on your own food ahead of time. That way, you won't be hungry and tempted to eat things you wouldn't normally, nor starved and in a rush to leave.

There is something to be said for making an exception every great once in a while, as well. As long as you can make the choice to indulge a bit without getting completely derailed, then go ahead and have a bite of the wedding cake, and go on to enjoy your otherwise healthy Paleo life.

# Resources

Where can you get more information or find online communities related to the Paleo Diet? Here is a list of resources consulted in the research of this book. Although this list is by no means exhaustive, it is a good place to get started on the Paleo lifestyle. Each resource contains more in-depth explanations and links to research about the Paleo Diet or related topics, as well as books, meal plans, videos, recipes, and more that you may find helpful.

Against All Grain: www.againstallgrain.com

- Website, blog, and cookbook by Danielle Walker with, as the title suggests, lots of information about how and why to eliminate grains and legumes from your diet, as well as lots of Paleo recipes.

Ancestor Approved: Paleo Gluten-free Recipes: www.paleoglutenfreerecipes.com

- Website and Paleo cookbooks by Tina Turbin

Ancestral Chef: www.ancestralchef.com

- Website with Paleo recipes, advice, meal plans, and entertaining how-to videos by Louise, "the ancestral chef."

Mark's Daily Apple: http://www.marksdailyapple.com

- Website, blog, and cookbooks by Mark Sisson based on his *The Primal Footprint* series with advice on the Paleo Diet as well as other healthy living tips including barefooting, sun exposure, and more.

Paleo Central: http://www.nerdfitness.com/paleo-central/

- A database and app created by Steve Kamb at www.nerdfitness.com that uses a very fun, conversational approach to learning about all things Paleo.

The Paleo Diet: www.paleodiet.com

- Touting itself as the original source for the diet plan by Dr. Loren Cordain, this website, blog, and accompanying cookbooks describes the diet in detail and gives a list of published research that back the science behind the diet, as well as offers (for a fee, of course) a Paleo meal plan subscription service.

The Paleo List: www.thepaleolist.com

- A website with the "Is It Paleo?" app by Cole Bradburn and Jim Lien, organized in question format with articles on all sorts of Paleo diet topics.

The Ultimate Paleo Guide: www.ultimatepaleoguide.com

- A website with articles, meal plans, recipes, a blog with multiple contributors and even a forum where you can find an online community of people practicing the Paleo lifestyle.